MOTHERPOWER AND INFANT FEEDING

AF804928

The University of Manchester
The John Rylands
University Library

MANCHESTER
1824

613.269
VAN

DYP6J

Motherpower and Infant Feeding

Penny Van Esterik

Zed Books Ltd
London

NLN/B GATE ✓ (DYP6J)

Motherpower and Infant Feeding was first published in paperback by Zed Books Ltd, 57 Caledonian Road, London N1 9BU, UK, and, under the title *Beyond the Breast-Bottle Controversy,* in cloth and paperback, by Rutgers University Press, 109 Church Street, New Brunswick, New Jersey 08901, USA, in 1989.

Copyright © Penny Van Esterik, 1989.

Cover designed by Robin Fox
Typeset by Huron Valley Graphics
Printed and bound in the United States
by/at BookCrafters, Chelsea, Michigan

All rights reserved

British Library Cataloguing in Publication Data

Van Esterik, Penny
Motherpower and infant feeding.
1. Babies. Feeding. Social aspects
I. Title
649'.3

ISBN 0-86232-886-1
ISBN 0-86232-887-X pbk

613.269
VAN

JOHN RYLANDS
UNIVERSITY
LIBRARY OF
MANCHESTER

To the memory of my mother

Elizabeth Brett Fair

And the promise of my daughter

Chandra Brett Van Esterik

CONTENTS

Foreword

JUST AS LAPPÉ AND COLLINS (1977) in *Food First* and George (1976) in *How the Other Half Dies* have taken the issue of malnutrition beyond amino acids and other nutrients to the underlying causes of malnutrition in an agriculturally productive world, so Penny Van Esterik in this book expands the breast-bottle controversy to issues related to poverty, the empowerment of women, the medicalization of infant feeding, and the commoditization of infant food. This book is both an extremely thoughtful case study and a new milestone in the literature on development.

That breastmilk is the only food, or fluid, human infants need to consume for the first four to six months of life is now widely accepted. It is no longer argued about by pediatricians, by multinational corporation executives, nor by breastfeeding advocates. But that was not always so. Almost a whole generation of American infants in the years after World War II were never breastfed.

Beyond the Breast-Bottle Controversy is a very important book.

The author takes a much written about topic and views it from an original set of angles; with perception she broadens the discussion and places it in the context of sustainable development. This volume should become essential (and enjoyable) reading for a broad range of individuals including all those concerned with urban and rural development in the nonindustrialized countries of the south; professionals and academics in various fields including health, sociology, anthropology, and development economics; many women exploring gender issues and feminism; those food industrialists and marketers involved in manufactured foods for infants and children; and lastly ordinary persons interested in how best to nurture babies.

In 1965 I wrote:

> It is most deplorable to see the cult of bottle feeding already taking grip on Africa. The immigrant community are of course to blame. What they do has often been regarded as sophisticated if not superior. But the commercial companies have not been slow to realize that there is money to be made out of this. . . . Advertising shows "how easy and how good" it is to bottle feed with such and such a product. For the majority of Africans, however, it is incredibly difficult and extremely bad. In fact commencement of bottle feeding is tantamount to signing the death certificate of many infants. The governments concerned should give serious thought to passing legislation to ban this type of advertising. . . . It cannot be overemphasized that human breastmilk is by far the best food for the human infant. In Tanzania it is estimated that 36,500,000 gallons of breastmilk are produced per year. The same quantity of cows milk at current retail prices would be worth over 9 million pounds ($40 million). (Latham 1965)

Two decades later I expressed myself this way:

> Among the factors that resulted in a greater use of bottle feeding in developing countries, two stand out as being of

> major importance, and both include practices that lend themselves to change. These are first the promotion of breastmilk substitutes by their manufacturers, particularly the multinational corporations, and second the failure of the health profession to advocate, protect and support breastfeeding. There is now overwhelming evidence of the health advantages of breastfeeding in terms of reduced infant morbidity and mortality when compared with artificially fed infants. . . . A relatively neglected major disadvantage of bottle feeding of infants is the serious economic consequences for poor families and nations. . . . Unfortunately however an increasing use of bottle feeding continues to be seen in many non-industrialized countries of the south. (Latham 1988)

What have we learned in the intervening twenty-three years between when those two pieces were written? Have we made any progress? In this fascinating new book, Penny Van Esterik provides some important answers to these questions. She achieves this by taking her analysis beyond the breast-bottle controversy.

To me, as a medical doctor and nutritionist concerned with good health and decent diets, with justice and equity for those living in poverty, the road ahead sometimes seems to have no end. I feel a little like those painting the Golden Gate Bridge across San Francisco Bay. By the time the painters reach the north shore, the south end of the bridge needs repainting. Penny Van Esterik would suggest that we should step back for a moment or two and consider the causes of the rust, the qualities of the paint, the structure of that magnificent bridge, and even the environment in which it stands.

There is now a large literature on the topic of infant feeding. There are good academic treatises, for example, *Human Milk in the Modern World* (1978) by the Jelliffes; there are interesting books by outspoken breastfeeding advocates, one of the best being Chetley's *The Politics of Baby Food* (1986); and there are helpful "how to" manuals such as *The Womanly*

Art of Breastfeeding by La Leche League (1976). But this excellent new book while academic is not a review of the scientific evidence; although it advocates breastfeeding and is critical of multinational corporations, it expounds a much broader form of advocacy than that found in other publications; and it is definitely not a manual on how to breastfeed successfully, although it does provide new insights on what needs to be done "to create conditions that make breastfeeding possible, successful, and valued in a given society."

This is the work of a scholar. The author is a distinguished anthropologist, but an unorthodox one. While taking an anthropological approach to her subject, she goes far beyond current anthropological thinking. In fact she appears to take some pleasure in criticizing her colleagues' expressed views that the infant formula controversy was irrelevant to anthropology.

As a woman, the author strongly believes that "infant feeding choices relate to the position and condition of women, ideologically and ecologically, in different societies." She cogently argues that infant feeding is a feminist issue, and that "the controversy helps us think through some of the most difficult dilemmas in feminist thought and action."

Penny Van Esterik has been an advocate for breastfeeding and against inappropriate formula use. With unusual candor she informs the reader of the personal experiences and influences that led her—a bottlefed baby—to become a breastfeeding mother and advocate. She states that "anthropologists have an important contribution to make to advocacy discourse for they are often the possessors of knowledge that can be used for change or stasis." She points out that "knowledge is not the problem" but that we are reluctant to use what is now known to improve the lot of women.

The author for four years worked with me at Cornell University as the anthropologist for a consortium of three institutions engaged in a large study of the determinants of infant feeding in four countries, namely Colombia, Kenya, Thailand, and Indonesia. I was the Principal Investigator at Cornell University for that study. Penny Van Esterik greatly broadened the scope of the investigation; she opened my eyes to new vistas and in uncountable ways enriched our understanding of infant feeding in these four countries. Her contribution cannot be measured. Her experience in the four cities of Bogotá, Nairobi, Bangkok, and Semarang has contributed substantially to this book. Only an ethnographer could select four women from some five thousand mothers in our study and so skillfully weave their lives into the rich fabric of a text that analyzes complex issues related to the most important questions of development and sustainability.

This book's major contribution lies in presenting a new view of an old controversy. The author really does go "beyond" the usual arguments pro and con formula feeding and devotes a major part of the text to a discussion of infant feeding in relation to the empowerment of women, the medicalization of the issue, and the commoditization of infant food.

She uses the controversy as a springboard to think through some of the major dilemmas in feminist thought and action; with surgical precision she dissects out the means used by doctors and health professionals (all too often assisted by industry) to bring infant feeding into their exclusive domain and to make an ordinary mammalian practice into a medical matter; and she clearly illustrates how both infant foods (breastmilk and formula) and their receptacles (breasts and feeding bottles) have become commodities to be promoted, marketed, and profited from, like any commercial good in the market place.

The final chapter in this book discusses the important connections between environmental concerns, empowerment of women, medicalization of life, commoditization of food, and the poverty environment. The conclusion surely is that we should be striving to improve the many conditions that effect the lives of women, rather than aiming our efforts mainly on infant feeding decisions. Conditions need to exist that make breastfeeding possible, desirable, enjoyable, and successful in all societies. To achieve this somewhat utopian situation, important international, and often national, changes are needed in current economic, social, and political conditions.

It is almost twenty-five years since I wrote:

> Anything that can be done to support breastfeeding is desirable. Human breastmilk is a most important protein-rich food. We must not in any respect be a party to seeing its disappearance, be it through advertising, through the creation of an aura that breastfeeding is a complicated difficult procedure, or through the fostering of the sort of breast culture that our society has developed. It is highly desirable that breastfeeding remains a natural normal procedure, and this may, I believe, be easier in places where the breast has not become a source of mystery, shame or pride. (Latham 1964)

As this book illustrates so well, we have won some battles. There has been considerable progress, but the ending of the Nestlé boycott and the increased prevalence of breastfeeding among affluent mothers in North America do not signal that a war has been won. Robert Chambers (1977) wisely suggests when discussing rural development that an important first step is for "professionals, the bearers of scientific knowledge, to step down off their pedestals, and sit down, listen and learn." This book will help us do just that.

Michael C. Latham
Professor of International Nutrition
Director, Program in International Nutrition
Cornell University, Ithaca, New York

Acknowledgments

IT IS A PLEASURE TO THANK those friends and colleagues who helped me think through many of the ideas expressed in this book. I would first like to express my gratitude to the project members participating in the infant feeding practices study (Contract AID/DSAN–C–0211): the project directors, Beverly Winikoff, Michael Latham, Giorgio Solimano, and all the consortium staff, particularly Jim Post, Virginia Laukaran, Mary Ann Castle, Terry Elliott, Somchai Durongdej, Thavisak Svetsreni, Moelyono Trastotenojo, Belen Semper de Paredes, Nico Kana, and Maria Eugenia Romero. Second, the steering committee of INFACT Canada provided me with constant encouragement to complete this project. I remain very dependent on the support and intellectual stimulation of many friends and colleagues whose advice and interest were critically important during the course of this work, in particular Bonnie Kettel, Cathy Campbell, Sheila Cosminski, Lenore Manderson, Margaret Kyenkya, and my students Carol Dignam, Annabel Sabloff, and Marilyn Walker. I owe a special thanks to Kathryn

Dettwyler for lending me her symposium title, "Beyond the Breast-Bottle Controversy."

I am most grateful to Pat Cates and the women in secretarial services at York University who transformed a mountain of yellow stickers into a finished manuscript. This book would undoubtedly never have been completed were it not for the encouragement of Marlie Wasserman who saw promise in a very ambitious prospectus and followed through with excellent support.

Finally, I thank my husband John Van Esterik who tolerated intolerable levels of snark and snarl during the preparation of this book because he believed in what I was doing and knew that one day it would be finished.

Motherpower and Infant Feeding

CHAPTER ONE

Introducing the Controversy

For most North Americans, the infant formula controversy is over. It ended with the lifting of the consumer boycott against Nestlé's products in October of 1984, ending one of the most successful consumer boycotts in history. Today, academics encourage scholars interested in infant feeding problems to go "beyond the breast-bottle controversy" and return to the "real" problems facing mothers in developing countries—poverty, powerlessness, hunger, and the unequal distribution of resources.

But for anthropologists, it is too soon to go far beyond the controversy. We need to move just far enough beyond it to provide a good angle for looking back at the events of the last decade (1975–1985) from a fresh perspective. For the infant formula controversy, or the breast-bottle controversy, is anything but a narrow activist cause: it raises some of the broadest and most significant questions of concern to anthropologists and other social scientists—questions concerning sustainable development, child survival, and the contradictions between research and advocacy modes of action. Although the boycott may be over and some advocacy groups may have chosen new concerns to bring to the public's attention, the problems associated with infant feeding have by no means disappeared, nor have the issues underlying the controversy become any simpler. But the voices are quieter, less strident, now that there is less need to shock or convert others. Among the many different voices, linked to differences in power and knowledge, are two, identified here as "advocacy discourse" and "research discourse." The popularity of the term "discourse" in current anthropological theory derives primarily from the works of Foucault (1980), Bourdieu (1984), and Geertz (1983). Often the term obscures more than clarifies. I use it here because it combines the concepts of conversation and spoken or written treatment of a subject with actions of understanding, reasoning, and turning over notions in the mind (Oxford English Dictionary 1971:430).

The silences after the controversy ceased to make newspaper headlines are revealing. It is as if the lessons learned from the controversy were only about power and exploitation, and not about lactation and nurturance. Lactation has no place in the report of the World Commission on the Environment and Development titled *Our Common Future* (1987), although sustainable development, the international economy, population, human resources, food security, energy, and industry—topics covered in the report—all relate to infant feeding choices. Lactation is also surprisingly absent from studies on women's health. The detailed index in *For Her Own Good* (150 years of experts' advice to women edited by Ehrenreich and English [1979]) has no entry for breast (between Marlon Brando and *Bride Magazine*), or lactation (between labor-saving appliances and *Ladies' Home Journal*). The recent book by Emily Martin, *The Woman in the Body,* has no index entries for breast, lactation, or infant feeding, although processes such as menstruation, childbirth, and menopause are treated in detail. Lactation as a process and breastmilk as a resource are again missing from the dominant discourses about development and women's health.

Underlying the infant formula controversy is a struggle over explaining change in infant feeding practices. This change is not so much a wholesale abandonment of breastfeeding as it is the addition of appropriate and inappropriate breastmilk substitutes and a related change in the interpretation of infant feeding. Health scientists try to define these changes by examining the rates of initiation, duration, or frequency of breastfeeding; anthropologists are more likely to try to explain how these changes occur. Shifts in patterns of infant feeding reflect three kinds of changes: (1) a change in the mode of feeding (e.g., from breastfeeding to bottle feeding); (2) a change in the product consumed (e.g., from breastmilk to other products); (3) a change in the interpretation of infant feeding.

Changes in the interpretation of infant feeding often include a shift from a process to a product orientation, with associated changes in social relations. Process models emphasize the continuity between pregnancy, birth, and the process of lactation rather than the product, breastmilk. The adoption of the biomedical model with its accumulated scientific evidence about the nutrient composition of breastmilk and breastmilk substitutes is a product-oriented model. The product interpretation is particularly compatible with the needs of the expanding market for breastmilk substitutes. Multinational pharmaceutical and food companies encourage the comparison between breastmilk and their industrial products. Both commoditization of infant foods and the medicalization of infant feeding encourage new kinds of social relations and new ways of thinking about infant feeding. The intention of this book is not to reargue the case for breastfeeding or provide new evidence incriminating the infant formula industry, but to situate the controversy more directly in current concerns about sustainable development, the empowerment of women, medicalization of infant feeding, and the commoditization of infant foods.

THE DEVELOPMENT OF THE CONTROVERSY

Advocacy Discourse

Since the mid-seventies, a broad range of people from all walks of life, most of them in North America and Europe, participated in a public debate known as the infant formula controversy. This controversy generated the largest support of any grass-roots consumer movement in North America, and its impact is still being felt in industry, governments, and citizen's action groups around the world. The most comprehensive history of the controversy is Chetley's, *The Politics of Baby Foods* (1986). Here, I trace the development of the controversy, highlighting the focal points of the social movement. An early presentation of the problem may be traced to an obscure Rotary Club address made by Dr. Cicely Williams in Singapore in 1939 entitled "Milk and Murder." She argued—perhaps to deaf ears—that the increase in morbidity and mortality in Singapore infants was directly attributable to the increase in bottle feeding with inappropriate breastmilk substitutes and the decline of breastfeeding (Williams 1986). Although conditions in other cities in the developing world may have been similar or worse than in Singapore, the voices of warning and reproach were hesitant, isolated, and easily ignored. Occasionally, reports from missionaries and health workers would confirm the devastating effects of this change on infant morbidity and mortality.

Since the thirties, the promotion of breastmilk substitutes has steadily increased, particularly in the urban markets of developing countries. In North America, competition between American pharmaceutical companies and the Depression reduced the number of companies producing infant formula to three large firms—Abbott (Ross), Bristol-Myers (Mead-Johnson), and American Home Products (Wyeth). Companies like Nestlé were already producing baby foods before the turn of the century. Both food- and drug-based companies producing infant formula expanded their markets during the post–World War II baby boom, as breastfeeding halved between 1946 and 1956 in America, dropping to 25 percent at hospital discharge in 1967 (Minchin 1985:216). By that time, the birthrate in industrialized countries had dropped, and companies sought new markets in the rapidly modernizing cities of developing countries.

As the industry magazines reported "Bad News in Babyland" in North America, their sales in developing countries increased, with only isolated and occasional protests from health professionals and consumer groups. One phrase in a speech caught the attention of a much wider audience. In 1968, Dr. Derrick Jelliffe labeled the results of the commercial promotion of artificial infant feeding as "commerciogenic malnutrition."

By the mid-seventies, publications like the *New Internationalist* (1973) were bringing the problem to public attention. Reports such as Muller's *The Baby Killer* (1974) and the German translation of the report titled *Nestlé Kills Babies* prompted responses from infant formula manufacturers. In 1974, Nestlé filed libel charges for five million dollars in a Swiss court against the Third World Action Group in Germany for their translation of *Nestlé Kills Babies,* leading to a widely publicized trial. Although the judge found the members of the group guilty of libel and fined them a nominal sum, he clearly recognized publicly the immoral and unethical conduct of Nestlé in the promotion of their products.

The libel suit and these sensationalist publications provided focal points around which public opinion gradually developed, strengthening the efforts of health professionals to establish policy guidelines on infant feeding through United Nation groups such as the Protein-Calorie Advisory Group. In North America, advocacy groups formed around the issue—most notably the Interfaith Center for Corporate Responsibility (ICCR), the Infant Formula Action Coalition (INFACT), and the International Baby Food Action Network (IBFAN). Formed in 1974, ICCR, monitored multinational corporations, provided information to church groups on responsible corporate investments, and publicized cases such as the lawsuit filed by the Sisters of the Precious Blood against Bristol-Myers in 1976 for misleading stockholders about their marketing practices. Although the case was dismissed, it did help to circulate more information about the marketing of breastmilk substitutes among groups interested in development and justice issues.

In 1977, other action groups coalesced to form INFACT and began the campaign to boycott Nestlé products in North America. The American INFACT grew out of study groups at the University of Minnesota, while the Canadian INFACT groups developed around justice ministries of the Anglican and United Churches. Later, IBFAN would draw these various coalitions together and represent the views of groups like INFACT, the Baby Milk Action Coalition in England, and the International Organization of Consumer Unions at international health policy conferences such as the World Health Assembly.

Groups like INFACT and ICCR made the North American public aware of the infant formula controversy (or the breast-bottle controversy) through an increasingly sophisticated campaign involving public debates, newsletters, radio and TV shows, petitions, demonstrations, posters, buttons, and a consumer boycott of Nestlé's products, which ended in 1984. Public education on the problem often featured the 1975 film,

Bottle Babies, a vivid portrayal of the tragic effects of bottle feeding in Kenya.

The advocacy position as defined by these groups is quite straightforward. It argues that the makers of infant formula should not be promoting infant formula and bottle feeding in developing countries where breastfeeding is prevalent and the technology for adequate use of infant formula is absent. Advocacy groups claim that multinational corporations (like Nestlé), in their search for new markets, launched massive and unethical campaigns, directed toward medical personnel and consumers, which encouraged mothers in developing countries to abandon breastfeeding for a more expensive, inconvenient, technologically complex, and potentially dangerous method of infant feeding—infant formula from bottles. For poor women who have insufficient cash for infant formula, bottles, sterilization equipment, fuel, or refrigerators; who have no regular access to safe, pure drinking water; and who may be unable to read and comprehend instructions for infant formula use, the results are tragic. Misuse of infant formula is a major cause of malnutrition and the cycles of gastroenteritis, diarrhea, and dehydration that eventually lead to death. Advocacy groups place part of the blame for this "commerciogenic malnutrition" on the multinational companies selling infant formula.

The infant formula companies responded to their critics by modifying their advertising to the public, but they were slow to meet all INFACT demands. It was never the intention of the advocacy groups to ban the sale of infant formula in developing countries, nor to pressure women to breastfeed, although their critics represented their aims in this light. The intention of INFACT is clearly stated in their demands:

1. An immediate halt to all promotion of infant formula
2. An end to direct promotion to the consumer, including mass-media promotion and direct promotion through

   posters, calendars, baby care literature, shows, wrist bands, and baby bottles
3. An end to the use of company "milk nurses"
4. An end to the distribution of free samples and supplies to hospitals, clinics, and homes of newborns
5. An end to promotion to the health professions and through health care institutions.

Nestlé's efforts were concentrated on trying to improve its tarnished public image by hiring a prestigious public relations firm, sending the clergy glossy publications about the company's contributions to infant health, and generally discrediting its critics as being merely uninformed opponents of the free enterprise system (Chetley 1986:46, 53).

Meanwhile, INFACT's campaign against the promotion of infant formula, begun in 1977, was extremely successful. In Toronto, for example, a market research firm found that 10 percent of the inhabitants of the city of two million were boycotting Nestlé products (INFACT Canada, Feb. 1982). The Toronto City Council not only endorsed the boycott but urged removal of Nestlé products from all civic premises.

The congressional hearings chaired by Edward Kennedy on the marketing and promotion of infant formula in the developing nations, in 1978, provided another focal point for American efforts. During the hearings, Ballarin, a manager of Nestlé's Brazilian operations, claimed to the amazement of the hearing that the boycott and the campaign against the infant formula companies were really an "attack on the free world's economic system," led by "a worldwide church organization with the stated purpose of undermining the free enterprise system" (United States Congress 1978:127). By 1979, continuing efforts by doctors like Jelliffe, Latham, and Hillman to bring the problem to the attention of health organizations, combined with the public efforts of the advocacy groups, convinced WHO that a code to regulate the marketing of infant formula should be drawn up. There is little doubt that the publicity and public pressure generated by advocacy groups through the Nestlé boycott were major factors in the convening of the WHO/UNICEF meetings in 1979, which resulted in the WHO Code of Marketing for Breastmilk Substitutes in 1981. In May 1981, the World Health Assembly adopted a nonbinding recommendation in the form of the WHO/UNICEF Code of Marketing for Breastmilk Substitutes, with a vote of 118 in favor, 3 abstentions, and the United States as the sole opposing vote. The code called on infant formula companies to halt mass advertising and direct marketing to mothers, to end the distribution of free samples and gifts to mothers, to stop using mothercraft nurses and health facilities to promote breastmilk substitutes, to end giving gifts and inducements to both retailers and health professionals, and to improve the labeling of their products, including specifying the superiority of breastmilk.

Following the establishment of the code, Nestlé publicly released special instructions to its marketing personnel to comply with the WHO Code and asked INFACT to call off the boycott. However, the boycott continued until 1984, because INFACT felt it was necessary to establish some means of monitoring company compliance with the code and that WHO member countries should draft national codes.

For all their rhetoric and their so-called confrontational tactics, the advocacy groups deserve great credit for bringing about what decades of clinical observations had failed to accomplish: public awareness and concern about infant formula abuse in developing countries. For the first time, nongovernmental organizations like INFACT and ICCR had a direct role in the deliberations at WHO and UNICEF in 1979; and their voices would be heard in subsequent meetings regarding infant feeding policy. Chetley points out that in spite of industry's concerns about the "scientific integrity" of allowing popular organizations and consumer groups to participate, delegates to the international meetings were impressed with the contributions of the nongovernmental organizations (1986:65–69). The advocacy groups turned a number of physicians into more outspoken public advocates for breastfeeding, stimulating a medical consensus on the value of breastfeeding. It was groups like IBFAN and INFACT that kept alive the underlying concern about corporate responsibility, human rights, and infant feeding as a justice issue.

The appeal of the infant formula controversy was due to the fact that it was presented as a simple, solvable, convergent problem. People were attracted to the campaign because it transformed many of their unspoken concerns into a clear, concrete example of exploitative behavior that could be acted upon. According to Schumacher (1977: 127), the more you study convergent problems, the more the answers converge; although some problems may remain unsolved at the moment, they are ultimately solvable. For many advocacy groups, the infant formula controversy was a convergent problem. The solution to the infant formula controversy was for multinational infant formula manufacturers to stop promoting infant formula in developing countries. When these companies agreed to abide by the conditions of the WHO/UNICEF Code of Marketing for Breastmilk Substitutes passed in 1981 and to meet some additional demands of the advocacy groups, then the boycott was lifted (Oct. 1984). For many supporters, this marked the end of the campaign—a victory of small grass-roots organizations over huge corporations. Like other convergent problems, when a solution was found, the entire issue ceased to be of further interest.

Research Discourse

Paralleling the advocacy campaign to limit the promotion of breastmilk substitutes in developing countries were a number of research projects on infant feeding. These research efforts were designed to provide more than anecdotal and clinical evidence regarding changes in infant feeding patterns. They were designed to measure patterns of infant feeding, their determinants, and their consequences. For example, in 1977, following Nestlé's widely publicized libel suit, the International Union of Nutrition Sciences (IUNS) undertook a collaborative study in Dar es Salaam (Tanzania), Colombo (Sri Lanka), and São Paulo (Brazil) to examine obstacles to breastfeeding and the marketing of baby foods. A larger collaborative study on breastfeeding was carried out by WHO in Chile, Ethiopia, Guatemala, India, Nigeria, the Philippines, Zaire, Hungary, and Sweden (WHO 1981). These studies provided descriptive statistics on patterns of infant feeding under different socioeconomic conditions and confirmed the extent of the marketing of industrially processed infant foods. The London-based World Fertility Surveys also contain information about breastfeeding. These surveys, in addition to country studies on infant feeding, suggest that although there was no shortage of information about infant feeding in developing countries, there were great differences about how to interpret the data. The accumulating research on infant feeding was funded by foundations, multilateral and bilateral development agencies, research institutes, and infant formula companies.

Following Senator Edward Kennedy's congressional hearings on the promotion of infant formula, the United States Agency for International Development (USAID) asked that proposals be submitted for the study of the determinants of infant feeding in developing countries. The contract was awarded to a consortium of Cornell and Columbia universities and the Population Council of New York under the direction of Dr. Beverly Winikoff, Dr. Michael Latham, and Dr. Giorgio Solimano. In 1980, I joined the interdisciplinary team as the consortium anthropologist.

The interdisciplinary study was conducted with research teams in four countries—Kenya, Colombia, Thailand, and Indonesia—using several different research methods. The study included a cross-sectional survey of mother-infant pairs from low- and middle-income areas; 980 from Nairobi (Kenya), 711 from Bogotá (Colombia), 1422 from Bangkok (Thailand), and 1356 from Semarang (Indonesia); marketing and medical infrastructure substudies; and community ethnographies. The study investigated the impact of a wide range of biological, social, cultural, and economic factors on infant feeding practices. The community ethnographies, although very brief, provided a basis for understanding the cultural context of infant feeding within a few households and neighborhoods in each city. I have used some of the study results to illustrate arguments throughout this book. The statistics cited come from the cross-sectional survey. The case studies developed in Chapter Two are based on the community ethnographies. After the research had been completed, a workshop for policy-makers was held to review the study results and make recommendations for improving infant feeding in each of the countries.

Site reports are available for each of the research sites from USAID. A major publication summarizes the results and provides a comparative analysis of different determinants of infant feeding (Winikoff et al. 1988). Study results are not summarized here, but the experience of participating in this research project informed many of the arguments developed in this book.

This study, like many other studies of infant feeding practices, demonstrates the complexity of the determinants of infant feeding patterns and hardly touches the controversy itself. The research studies confirmed what even the most radical advocates knew in their heart of hearts—that the basis for mothers' infant feeding decisions is not at all simple and straightforward. Promotion and advertising of infant formula are factors that cannot always be unambiguously demonstrated statistically. The determinants of infant feeding patterns are multifaceted, complex, and poorly understood. There was indeed a problem concerning the increasing use of breastmilk substitutes, but this was not one of Schumacher's convergent problems. Instead, the research on infant feeding epitomized a divergent problem that defied a simple solution. Even the partial answers emerging from research appear to contradict one another and spin the problem solver in opposite directions. Divergent problems cannot be solved; rather, they must be grappled with over and over again, like many human problems anthropologists explore. Their importance lies not in their outcome but in the process of interpretation and reinterpretation they require.

Explaining why mothers shift from breastfeeding to bottle feeding with infant formula is just such a divergent problem. Each of the explanations emerging from research results—women's formal employment, mothers' illness, the stresses of urban living, the health care delivery system, marketing practices of infant food manufacturers, among others—offers partial answers that do not simply converge or diverge. They often avoid addressing the issues raised by the advocacy discourse altogether. In fact, the advocacy discourse and the research discourse offer very different frameworks for interpreting the infant formula controversy.

Geertz refers to these contrasting modes of discourse as "blurred genres" (1983:20). In the infant formula controversy, the loudest and clearest discourses are the advocacy, corporate, and research discourses. The text analogy that Geertz develops is particularly apt for the infant formula controversy. The advocacy and corporate texts developed as a reaction to each other, each providing commentaries and "translations" to make the text "readable" for the other. Corporate analysis of advocacy arguments and advocacy analysis of corporate arguments provide critiques that make each side more understandable to the other and offer the public an opportunity to assess the worth of both arguments. These critiques passed back and forth in memos clarifying the "facts and fallacies" in the two positions. The research discourse is not based on an analysis of either the corporate or the advocacy text, but instead purports to present objective truth, presumably ready for use by either advocacy or corporate supporters. However, the interaction between advocacy, corporate, and research perspectives is important to note since research is more often funded, directly or indirectly, by corporate groups than by advocacy groups. This is not to say that research funded by pharmaceutical or food companies marketing breastmilk substitutes and supplementary foods is deliberately falsified, but rather that funding sources influence the kinds of questions asked and interpretations made. It is becoming more and more difficult to find funding for infant feeding research and publication that is not tied directly or indirectly to industry interests. As one colleague said with a smile, "if we can't criticize industry, we may as well shut up shop . . . as long as you don't say Nestlé kills babies, because we've got Nestlé money in the department." What is significant is what does not get researched, what questions are not asked.

The contradictions emerging from the juxtaposition of the advocacy discourse and the research discourse occur at two levels simultaneously: first, at the level of understanding the infant feeding decisions of mothers in developing countries, and second, at the level of the controversy itself. For example, health professionals influence mothers' decisions about infant feeding and are also actors or potential actors in the breast-bottle controversy. This poses a particular dilemma for linking knowledge about infant feeding to social action about infant feeding.

It is these complexities and contradictions that suggest that the infant formula controversy is really about many things in addition to infant feeding. It is embedded in a number of other submerged discourses, all of which have their own agendas and priorities. This book examines some of these other processes in an attempt to discover how they have affected our interpretation of the infant formula controversy and our resulting social action (or inaction). The breast-bottle controversy is also about poverty environments, empowerment of women, medicalization of infant feeding, and commoditization of food. The controversy and the social action it generated still continue, but many activities, like monitoring and writing reports, are more routinized now. It is time to reflect on how some of these broader debates are related in different ways to the controversy. In many ways, the controversy is a paradigmatic case for thinking through these four themes.

Poverty Environments. The infant formula controversy is seldom viewed as part of the problem of renewable resources and environmental conditions. The problems about appropriate resource utilization are most apparent in the households of the urban poor, where environmental conditions impinge directly on infant morbidity and mortality. Households face problems of shared, expensive, impure, and undependable water supplies, expensive fuel, few refrigerators, and competing demands on scarce and irregular cash incomes. Environmental conditions and perpetual poverty determine how women establish priorities for infant and child feeding. Infant feeding decisions must be understood in the context of these poverty environments. Environmental conditions, then, become key to improving infant health. The patterns of infant feeding, which appear to be personal choices or culturally patterned, can also be tied to the institutions of the world system.

Environmental issues pervade the infant formula controversy. Water pollution, nitrosamines in feeding teats and pacifiers, and chemical pollutants in breastmilk are all symptoms of changing environment conditions in developed as well as developing countries. From an environmental perspective, the controversy raises the following question: what are the consequences of replacing a perfectly adapted renewable resource with a non-renewable resource requiring high energy expenditure and producing waste—wasted products, wasted energy, wasted money, and wasted lives?

Empowerment of Women. Women's control over their own lives and bodies has much to do with the choices available to them for infant feeding. Their access to food, flexibility in scheduling and work load, and social support system influence their management of lactation or their decision to bottle feed. Ultimately, infant feeding choices relate to the position and condition of women, ideologically and economically, in different societies.

At the level of the controversy, it is interesting and surprising to find the lack of a consistent feminist position on the infant formula controversy. Examination of conservative, liberal, radical, and socialist feminist arguments helps explain the contradictions and the strange coalitions that formed during the controversy. The advocacy position was supported more by individual women than women's groups. But "feminist rhetoric" serves infant formula companies well in promoting bottle feeding in both developed and developing countries ("liberation in a can"). While western feminist arguments are seldom adequate in developing countries, it is nonetheless important to understand how women's groups and feminist groups in different countries define the issues related to infant feeding.

Medicalization of Infant Feeding. Infant feeding is increasingly seen as part of the medical domain and the responsibility of health professionals in both developed and developing countries. How has this been accomplished? And how has medicalization affected infant feeding decisions of mothers in developed and developing countries? Certainly, attitudes of health professionals and hospital routines have had a substantial impact on how mothers think about infant feeding alternatives. For example, how does the doctor's advice to stop breast-feeding affect individual mothers? What is the relation between health care facilities and the infant formula industry? How does the medical model in developing countries interact with the personal models mothers use to decide how to feed their infants? These competing models must be examined in relation to the position and condition of women through women's dependence on medical expertise.

Throughout the controversy, medical testimonies and endorsements were sought by all sides to defend their arguments. Expert medical knowledge became the established standard for defining research priorities. The devaluation of women's knowledge of infant feeding is a key argument in analyzing the production of knowledge for social action.

Commoditization of Infant Food. The use of infant formula, processed weaning foods, and feeding bottles reflects the adoption of many western foods in developing countries. The problem of bottle feeding, then, is embedded in the processes of delocalization and prestige emulation of food in developing countries. How do food products develop socially sustained sign values? To what extent has bottle feeding become a status symbol? Certainly, advertising is implicated, but how potent is it? Is the consumer demand for western foods already there or is it created by promotion? The adoption of commercial infant foods is not only a question of taste and technology transfer but also of who controls the information necessary for successful technology transfer.

The role of infant food manufacturers in the breast-bottle controversy is well documented. Manufacturers had to protect their interests and expand their markets while fending off their critics. There are parallels with other cases of food delocalization encouraged by multinational corporations as they expand their markets in developing countries.

An examination of these four themes shows that the breast-bottle controversy is far from over. Until these and other related issues are addressed, many questions will remain unanswered. Once we have examined these four themes underlying the controversy, the arguments must be reconstructed to give a coherent picture of the relations between them. In Bateson's terms, we seek the "pattern that connects" these divergent perspectives in the concluding chapter.

REFLECTIONS

These themes have not emerged by chance nor have they been developed from careful deductive logic about infant feeding, although both chance and logic played a part. The choice of discourses and the problems posed by advocacy action reflect my personal experiences with infant feeding and with the controversy. While it is tempting to feign detachment and objectivity about the topic, such a stance is contrary to the theoretical position underlying this book. If I hope to be able to reconcile the discourses underlying the controversy, I must also place myself as the instrument of analysis under scrutiny. What follows, in Geertz's terms, is the "systematic unpackings" of my conceptual world (1983:22). The breast-bottle controversy brought to light many personal dilemmas for women who supported or rejected the advocacy argument, or attempted to distance themselves entirely from the issue. The breastfeeding experience is so personal and intimate that it evokes passionate and often sentimental emotional responses in women. Decisions not to breastfeed or to breastfeed but only briefly or reluctantly evoke equally strong feelings. In this section, I identify my personal biases on this issue in case any of them might remain undetected by the last page. My life experiences have influenced my interpretation of infant feeding research, the infant formula controversy, and therefore the construction of the book's argument.

My mother's recollections about breastfeeding were all negative. Stories of bleeding nipples, hot poultices, binding cloths, swollen, pus-filled breasts, and bad smells contrasted with stories of heroic (and probably exaggerated) wartime efforts to obtain enough rationed supplies to prepare elaborate formula made from Farmer's Wife evaporated milk, corn syrup, and lactic acid milk for me. Breastfeeding attempts—all failures—nearly killed my mother, to hear her tell the tale. I thought very little about infant feeding until I was pregnant. I doubt that I had seen more than one or two breastfeeding mothers in my life. But the times were ripe for experimentation. I was away from home in graduate school in the Midwest in a town where childbirth classes, infants in back carriers, the La Leche League, and yogurt and granola were the norm. After prenatal classes and a La Leche League meeting where I saw more breastfeeding in two hours than I had seen throughout my life, I decided to breastfeed.

As I remember, financial considerations were foremost in my mind. I almost resented the "earth-mother" commitment of many homebound breastfeeding mothers I met. Chandra was born in early September, the week before lectures began and three months before my doctoral exams were scheduled. Somehow, I decided to breastfeed without any thought about how to balance graduate work and infant care. My mother, who stayed with us for the first month, was a great help with infant care but was unable to offer any breastfeeding advice: in fact, I think she felt extremely sorry for me beginning this painful duty. The first few weeks I needed assistance from experienced nursing mothers on general management problems (and to restrain my mother who accepted the hospital's gift pack of ready-to-serve Similac, a product she found very impressive).

Over the months, I became more emotional about breastfeeding and found it the most pleasant part of a hectic routine of studying, teaching, and preparing for exams. I alternated breastfeeding on demand with occasional substitute bottles of infant formula, with no ill effects for mother or daughter. I doubt that I could have combined the demands of breastfeeding and graduate school had I not used occasional substitute bottles of infant formula. As I recall, I stayed with Similac, the brand in the hospital gift pack. A pediatrician who was unusually supportive of breastfeeding followed Chandra's development with interest, particularly because she failed to develop the family allergies. Since we planned fieldwork in Thailand, we kept Chandra breastfeeding for sixteen months to take her (and us) over the hurdles of international travel in Asia, uncertain water supplies, and settling into Bangkok and rural Thai life.

Perhaps I had smug satisfaction at easing some difficult life circumstances by breastfeeding, but I was still uncomfortable with much of the pro-breastfeeding rhetoric and unaware of the extent to which my decision had been made in a bottle feeding world. The broader implications of breastfeeding in a bottle feeding world were brought home to me in Thailand, in 1973, when a Thai pediatrician pressured me to take samples of Lactogen for my daughter who, at about thirteen months, was putting away an astounding amount of Thai food in addition to breastmilk. She developed diarrhea after drinking reconstituted full cream milk for a few days. The pediatrician blamed breastmilk for her diarrhea, advised me to stop breastfeeding immediately, and suggested I begin giving her Lactogen in a bottle. This experience, combined with increased contact with Bangkok professional women who found breastfeeding repugnant, alerted me to the rapidly changing attitudes toward infant feeding in Thailand, later developed in papers on the subject (Van Esterik 1977, 1982).

The advocacy arguments against the infant informula manufacturers, which began appearing in the mid-seventies, made a great deal of sense to me, and I began to follow the ICCR and INFACT campaigns. When I was a student, I participated in civil rights marches, anti-nuclear power demonstrations, and protests against the war in Southeast Asia. As a "weekend protester," I was easily swept along with current concerns, often without a full critical understanding of the issues. In the late seventies I accepted invitations to discuss my Thai experiences with church groups struggling to decide whether to join the Nestlé boycott or support shareholder's resolutions against companies like Bristol-Myers. In the late seventies, in my first full-time teaching position, I was criticized by anthropology colleagues for "getting involved," and "losing my objectivity."

I was disturbed by criticism from anthropologists, who objected to the advocacy rhetoric I would use in public debates. However, I was more disturbed by my colleagues' lack of interest; they would cite many anecdotes from their own fieldwork supporting the advocacy position, but they found the advocacy campaign itself of no professional concern to anthropologists. When I found myself debating anthropologists who represented Nestlé or other infant formula companies, I became more discouraged. One of my more painful lessons occurred during the 1980 annual business meeting of the American Anthropological Association when a graduate student called for a resolution of support for the work of INFACT and the WHO/UNICEF Code. Like a chicken-hearted coward, I kept quiet on the advice of a colleague who urged me not to look like a radical student by taking a public stand on an issue that would probably be defeated. The resolution was effortlessly defeated with arguments such as "the evidence is not all in."

Yet that same meeting voted support for a series of equally undocumented resolutions.

This experience underscored for me the disjunction of the advocacy and research discourses within academia and resulted in a paper on whether the infant formula controversy had any relevance to anthropology (Van Esterik 1980a). It was student response to this issue that lead me to conclude that the controversy should be of concern to anthropology. The controversy occasionally crept into my classes on human evolution, sex roles, and applied and nutritional anthropology. By bringing the issue into anthropology classes, I began to see the variety of topics that needed to be examined before the issue could be fully understood.

The opportunity to explore those topics came when I joined the consortium to study the determinants of infant feeding in developing countries. At Cornell University, I learned much more about the health and nutritional consequences of bottle feeding and the complexities behind research designs and causal relationships. Having learned the research discourse, I lost the strident advocate's voice that allowed me comfortably to oversimplify the issues during public debates. Much later, I wrote of the experience of wearing the "wrong hat"; I "spoke research" when I should have "spoken adovcacy" in a debate with a very sophisticated team from Nestlé (Van Esterik 1986a). Although my research writing resulted in the loss of the theatricality and rhetoric necessary for advocacy discourse, I was complimented by a colleague in medical anthropology who said that as my work became more objective and unemotional, it became stronger. I lived with the contradictions between advocacy and research discourse without fully recognizing the importance of this disjunction for theoretical issues in anthropology.

The infant feeding study provided an opportunity to see firsthand how infant formula is promoted in developing countries, yet how inadequate our analytical capacities are to demonstrate watertight cause-and-effect relations between promotion and infant feeding decisions. I was occasionally frustrated when I found myself contributing to the project by writing more narrow papers on breastfeeding and women's work (Van Esterik and Greiner 1981) and insufficient milk (Greiner et al. 1981; Van Esterik 1988). What stands out from the experience of traveling back and forth to the four countries and working with the ethnographers are several incidents that had no place in these more objective papers I was writing. In Bogotá, I remember the anger of one ethnographer when she explained that among the few poor households she was working with, one infant was fully breastfed (her "blue-ribbon baby") and was healthy and developing well, while another infant was skinny and sickly and receiving watered-down infant formula—and how important this difference would be in her analysis. But she returned one day to find that the breastfed baby had died of a respiratory infection after a brief bout of measles. Even breastfeeding was not enought to protect the child from the cold, damp air blowing through the shack. I had no answer for her grief and anger and could only file away a painful lesson. And in Thailand, the apology of a poor women who said she could not afford anything good for her baby, and so she had to breastfeed. It was on that visit that I really listened to the phrasing of the research questions in Thai; the question literally asks what kind of Lactogen do you feed your baby? How firmly certain brand names become part of the language, unconsciously, insidiously. What are the processes that make us unable to think in the generic and think first of the brand? In Semarang, I remember the ethnographer who was supposed to be recording the infant feeding practices in her assigned household. But because the family was not able to afford suitable food for the children, she began to "smuggle" fresh fruit to the family and worried that the consortium anthropologist would "catch" her unscientific behavior. Less poignant, but more revealing, was the weekend "off" in Nairobi. I was going to go to a game park, but learned that some of the consortium staff and others actively involved in infant feeding issues were going to examine a draft of the proposed Kenyan National Code on the marketing of breastmilk substitutes. The draft looked at first glance like the WHO/UNICEF Code. But after cutting all the sentences into clauses and rearranging them, the staff found that the phrasing resembled the ICIFI "code" proposed by the International Council of Infant Food Industries. It required a lawyer's sharp eye to catch the shifts in language. The long day resulted in a detailed critique of the draft, which suggested changes that would make the Kenyan national code meet the spirit and letter of the of the WHO/UNICEF Code. Ironically, INFACT Canada is currently involved in an identical task. In October 1987, Health and Welfare Canada accepted a new industry code on the marketing of breastmilk substitutes, produced by CIFA (Canadian Infant Formula Association), which is much weaker than the WHO/UNICEF Code.

These experiences brought me a degree of wisdom and understanding that was not reflected in my research reports. Perhaps my work on infant feeding style (Van Esterik 1985a,b) was a response to the research discourse on infant feeding and my discomfort with writing in the style of health sciences. I found myself wanting to write of meaning, analogies, and hegemony rather than variables, frequencies, and causation.

The completion of the study in 1984 coincided with the ending of the Nestlé boycott. The juxtaposition of these two events radicalized me more than the INFACT debates or the study results. For in spite of the success of the campaign to limit the promotion of infant formula in developing countries and the volume of computer printouts from the study, the sale of infant formula continues to increase. As the processes underlying the changes in infant feeding practices become more clearly understood, marketing practices shift to take advantage of new opportunities—specialized infant formula here, closer relations with nursing schools there.

Since returning to full-time teaching in anthropology, I have reflected upon how the infant formula controversy is embedded in the broader processes of medicalization and the commoditization of food in developing countries. It was not until I began to view the issue in a broader political economy framework that I began to understand more about my early discomfort with the "earth-mother" model of breastfeeding and to explore feminist approaches to the controversy. I now use the knowledge gained from these experiences related to the infant feeding controversy to help interpret other issues related to food, women, and third world development. And in spite of my colleagues who said the infant formula controversy was (a) too narrow, and (b) irrelevant to anthropology, I delight in returning to a discipline broad and flexible enough to embrace such small matters.

CHAPTER TWO

Poverty Environments

IN THIS CHAPTER, I want to describe how four women from four very different urban communities are connected to processes and institutions that crosscut national boundaries. These processes and institutions, part of the broader world system, can affect women's infant feeding decisions in many different ways. In the course of ethnographic fieldwork, it is tempting to dwell on the uniqueness of individual lives and the particular events in communities and to disregard the broader connections between communities. Yet these connections are important for understanding how particular households and communities in third world countries are integrated into the world system. They are also important reminders of the links between "us" and "them," a particularly important aspect of the infant formula controversy. For it was through advocacy action that many women in North American cities came to appreciate the difficulties poor women face in raising their children.

Over one billion people live in cities—a tenfold increase from 1920 (World Commission on Environment and Development

1987:16). But many of these cities have not been able to provide their rapidly growing numbers with the services and facilities necessary to maintain an adequate quality of life for them and for their children. In Nairobi, Bangkok, and Bogotá this has resulted in the creation of illegal settlements with even cruder facilities than in the areas of legal settlement. These four women live under conditions of environmental stress, with deficiencies in housing, water, sanitation, and often basic food security. Poverty pollutes their environment.

Four Women

Rosa, Grace, Sunoto, and Amporn were participants in the ethnographic component of the four-country infant feeding practices study introduced in Chapter One. The life stories of these four women were developed by teams of ethnographic researchers in each of the four countries. The teams chose three or four low-income neighborhoods in their respective cities and spent about three months in intensive participant observation in the communities and households; they interviewed on topics such as household composition, physical setting, mother's activities, community resources, and infant feeding practices. Their analyses and case studies provided background for the construction of the infant feeding survey in each city.

Why choose these four women? The reasons are arbitrary and opportunistic. The ethnographers in the four cities took particular care in writing up the cases of these women—perhaps because they saw in their lives certain themes repeated throughout the study, perhaps because more of a human connection was made. Something in their lives touches the lives of the ethnographers. Perhaps it is a personal response on my part, since I met three of them; I sat in their homes and could therefore picture their circumstances more clearly. But they are in no way atypical. Their neighbors could equally well illustrate the conditions of life in these communities.

If they could meet, they would have much in common in spite of the great geographical and cultural differences separating them. Rosa from the southeast corner of Bogotá in the foothills of the Andes; Grace from Kibera, a shantytown stretching west of Nairobi; Sunoto from the residential suburbs west of Semarang, Central Java; and Amporn from an old established district of Dhonburi, Bangkok.

Rosa. Rosa Suarez was born in Santander (near the Venezuela border), the seventh child of eight in her family. Her father died when she was two years old. She never went to school but learned to write her name and read a little. When she was eleven, she went to live with relatives in the town of Bucaramanga until she was sixteen, when she went alone to live in Bogotá. For two years she worked as a domestic in families' homes and then met a man with whom she lived for seven years. Throughout these years, she had worked in various homes during the day, doing housework and caring for children. When the ethnographers met Rosa, she had one child five years old and a set of male twins aged seven months.

Before the twins were born, her circumstances worsened: "During the pregnancy I was poorly fed, at times with soup and brown sugar water. When my husband learned that we were going to have twins, we had a fight and he left. In the seventh month I began to hemorrhage, perhaps because of fighting with him, and I went to the hospital. There, the doctor gave me a pill to calm me and said that the children must be delivered or they will probably die. They gave me a tranquilizer and took out the babies with forceps. I was not expecting them so soon and I had nothing ready for them. Also, I did not have the means for raising them. The doctor proposed to me that I give him one of my children since he and his wife always wanted to have one and could not. I told him, never—that I wasn't capable of giving away a child, and I would find a way of taking care of them. When I left the hospital, they recommended to me that I make a sack out of rags and fill it with bottles of hot water to keep the children from dying of cold." Rosa survived these difficult times because of the care and advice she received from women for whom she worked.

Rosa's shack consists of two tiny rooms, one containing a table and a bed in which everyone sleeps. The other room serves as a kitchen, pantry, and bathroom. There is no plumbing in her house, but she can get as much water as she needs from her neighbors. She prepares food in a single dish on a two-burner hot plate. She has a few pans and utensils, but she had to sell her pressure cooker when the babies became sick. Rosa's economic situation is critical. She works sporadically, washing clothes for neighbors, and is paid in food or money. She works only about four days per week because she does not always have a place to leave the babies.

Rosa herself was breastfed for two years and then was fed goat's milk because it was considered healthier than cow's milk. Sometimes they drank milk from burros, but it was so heavy that some children could not digest it. They also ate other foods such as sugar cane juice, corn cakes, yuca, plantains, meat, calabash, oranges, and blackberries. Fruits and vegetables were given to the children as soon as they were able to grasp them.

Rosa's method of feeding her oldest child was very different from the way she was fed. He was breastfed for the first two months; then Rosa caught a fever that affected her milk production. After that he was given "Dutch milk," eggs, juice, fruit, vegetables, and meat. The older child ate well because Rosa's companion made enough money. The twins, on the other hand, were born just after he left and did not receive the same good food. Because they were born prematurely, Rosa was completely unprepared for them. The doctor advised her to breastfeed them as much as she could, but she had already realized that breastfeeding was the only practical method of feeding. She felt as though she were feeding one or the other all day long. When they were not full, she supplemented with S-26 infant formula. She also gave them bottles of sugar water with four spoonfuls of milk added. At five months, Rosa gave the twins other food because they looked ill. Little by little, she introduced egg yolk, guava juice, and vegetable soup, all specially prepared for them. But their meals depended entirely upon whether Rosa had any money for food or was given any food at work that day.

Rosa noticed that one of the twins ate more than the other and was more alert. Both babies were frequently sick with bronchitis, grippe, stomach problems, and the like, which made it very difficult for Rosa to leave them in a nursery to go to work. Any food she could get was given to the twins because she felt the older child was well fed at nursery school. If she had extra food, she would feed her older child at night. Rosa ate at her neighbor's home in exchange for cleaning or babysitting.

The hospital where the twins were born sponsored talks reinforcing the importance of breastmilk. At the health center, advice on vegetables and fruits was offered. The nuns at the nursery school provided milk when possible. Rosa depends almost entirely upon friends and neighbors for such things as food, baby-sitting, jobs, and clothing. Rosa is only minimally exposed to advertising. She has a radio that she does not listen to and sees a newspaper occasionally at a neighbor's home. She is not impressed with "modern" foods.

Rosa learned from her mother at an early age how to use herbs for infant care. She feeds herbs to her children, baths them in herbs, uses compresses from herbs, and generally relies on them to cure most ailments. Rosa is also careful about the difference between hot and cold foods. “Hot people should not eat cold foods and cold people should not eat hot foods.” She values soup because “it makes more blood, particularly when it is made from carrots and greens.” She believes that fried food is not good for babies or adults because the oil is bad for the stomach. Rosa considers a bottle with water and sugar cane juice (*panela*), to be very good because “panela provides calories whereas sugar is just a sweetener.” Rosa feels that breastmilk is best because “the babies are tranquil.”

Rosa is in no way constrained by her “traditional” ideas about infant feeding. Her constraints are clearly financial; her living conditions are totally inadequate—the cold, damp mountain air blows through the flimsy walls of the shack, chilling Rosa’s body and soul and reducing her will to struggle for her infant sons.

Grace. Grace was twenty-six when the ethnographers met her in the shantytown of Kibera, Nairobi. Her living conditions, like Rosa’s, are inadequate, and she struggles for the most basic resources for herself and her three daughters. She grew up near Siaya in western Kenya and still has access to three acres of land. She dreams of leaving Nairobi and returning there when she can persuade her husband to seek employment away from Nairobi.

Grace had more education than Rosa, but her family did not have money to send her to secondary school. Like Rosa, she came to the city as a housemaid and later eloped with her husband. The family lives in a one-room house at the end of a block of rooms. The walls are roughly constructed of mud; there is a small window in one of the walls and a door made of wood. Garbage and litter are scattered all over the grass directly in front of the house. There is no bathroom, but the family bathes after dark outside their room. There is one pit latrine nearby, which is used by about twelve households. Tap water is sold at kiosks where each can of water costs about four cents. The family uses four cans a day for cooking and drinking. Grace gets water for bathing and washing clothes from a stream near the Nairobi Dam. For her, clean water is an expensive, precious commodity.

Grace's first daughter was born in 1978. She breastfed the baby for four months and then stopped because there was no milk. The child cried after breastfeeding. She developed measles at eight months, but had no other health problems. Grace's second baby born in 1980, was breastfed for three months, after which she refused the breast because there was no milk. The baby pulled hard on the nipples, but nothing came out. Her youngest daughter was seven months old when the ethnographers met her.

Grace started attending a prenatal clinic at six months because she needed to be "booked in" or she could not be delivered in the hospital. Grace learned many new ideas at the clinic about a balanced diet and what to prepare for the new baby. But it turned out that her baby was born at home with the assistance of a neighbor. The neighbor was not an expert, but she had helped many other women in the village. Although she does not charge any fee, she is given small presents. Grace had to deliver at home because her husband had returned to his rural home, leaving her with the young children. Going to the hospital would have meant leaving the children alone in the house. The baby slept beside Grace immediately after delivery and continues to do so. The baby was given boiled water shortly after birth, and Grace continued to give her glucose water for two days because she had no milk at all. She boiled water, and when it was cool enough, she added one teaspoonful of glucose to about four ounces of water and gave it to the baby, using a big cup and a spoon, imitating her previous hospital delivery experience.

The baby cried constantly for the first two months, waking

JOHN RYLANDS
UNIVERSITY
LIBRARY OF
MANCHESTER

her up five times in the night. She had no problem with getting the infant to breastfeed, but believed her milk was not enough. She had to give supplementary feeds very early and gave glucose water after every breastfeed.

She took her daughter to the clinic two months after delivery and was advised to give supplementary milk feeds. She then bought S-26 at U.S. $2.73 for a small can and started giving this as she had been instructed at the clinic. Twice a day (10 A.M. and 9 P.M.) she gave S-26 in addition to breastmilk and glucose water. When the baby was three months old, a neighbor suggested she give her some porridge twice in a day, as that might settle the baby down in the night. She made porridge from white maize meal and added sugar and some drops of lemon juice.

She continued with S-26, porridge, and glucose water, each given twice a day. She stopped buying S-26 and glucose because the baby was big enough to take fresh cow's milk in a packet. Also, buying S-26 and glucose was making a big demand on the family's small income. She was breastfeeding the baby on demand, but there was just a little milk left.

When the baby was five months old, she developed thick crops of rashes on her body, severe red sticky eyes, a sore mouth, and a dirty tongue. She took her to the clinic, where the child was given good attention and the illness diagnosed as measles. She gave her medicine for three days but did not notice any improvement and therefore decided to take her child to Kenyatta National Hospital where the baby was admitted to the Paediatric Observation Ward with severe dehydration and post-measles bronchio-pneumonia. Grace and the baby were in this ward for four days. The baby was fed intravenously and treated for marasmus. When her daughter improved, Grace arranged for a public health nurse to see her home in Kibera, and then she was discharged with a pound of dried skim milk powder.

Back at home, she wakes daily at 6 A.M. to make breakfast for her husband. If there is no milk left from the previous day, she makes porridge from only white maize meal. At 7 A.M. Grace sends her eleven-year-old helper to buy two liter packets of milk from the kiosk. The other children have tea with milk and bread if available. Porridge is made for the youngest child and a little milk is added to it if there is any.

The young helper collects water from the stream, lights the charcoal brazier, and helps bathe the younger children while Grace is busy with the baby. Grace settles the baby to sleep by about 8 A.M. By then she has finished sweeping the house and has made the bed. The other children's sleeping mat and blankets are spread outside in the sun. Her helper washes the baby's linen and spreads the washing out on the grass to dry. Grace gives the baby glucose water or milk at about 11 A.M. The milk is warmed and given by bottle, which was rinsed with warm water after the first porridge feed.

Since her husband does not come home for lunch, Grace makes lunch for the children and herself at about 12.30 P.M. If they are eating fish or meat with porridge, the youngest is given mashed porridge with soup and is then given five ounces of warm milk. At about 4 P.M. her helper makes porridge for the whole family. Grace serves the children the porridge and keeps some for her husband. She prepares a little of the porridge for the youngest, adding lemon juice and sugar to the porridge in the bottle. At about 5 P.M. she puts on the fire for the evening meal and collects her second container of water from the water seller. Her helper collects more water from the stream for bathing herself and the other children.

Twice a week, Grace leaves very early in the morning for the wholesale vegetable market in Nairobi and returns by bus and on foot by about 10 A.M. Outside the house, she sets up her vegetable stall and sells onions, tomatoes, greens, and occasionally dried fish and groundnuts to her neighbors. She would like to sell at her stall near the main road, where she would get more buyers, but since her youngest child's illness, she sells only in front of her house.

The two older children have large round bellies, brown hair, and signs of kwashiorkor and scabies infection. These children and her helper stay outside most of the time, playing with their peer groups in the village. The young children use the space behind the house for a toilet. The helper then has to pick up all the feces with pieces of paper and put them down the public toilet.

Like Rosa, Grace's attitudes were influenced by the woman for whom she worked as a maid. She has also been influenced by the hospital staff and some of her close women friends. The whole family goes to church every Sunday and buys new clothes once a year before Christmas. If Grace had the money, she dreams of being able to give her youngest the best possible diet: "S-26, Cerelac, Ribena (a black currant syrup), glucose, cod liver oil, eggs, meat, fish, and fruits." But for Grace, these foods are beyond her means.

Sunoto. In the western suburbs of Semarang, Central Java, Ibu Sunoto, twenty-five years old, raises her two children, a boy, six years, and a girl, eighteen months. She was born in Surabaya, the third of seven sisters. When she was fourteen, she started work at a printing office and stayed there for five years. When she was nineteen, she was introduced to her sister's friend and two months later they married.

Her husband is a truck driver from Semarang, and they speak Javanese at home. Her husband goes to work at 9 A.M. and comes back at night. She takes care of her children and does the cooking, shopping, and washing every day. She plans to send their first child to elementary school when he is seven, but she has not made plans for the second child yet because she is too young. She does not have any other work activities but her housework. She does not take part in any local women's groups because she is "ashamed and believes she has no ability."

For three years, Sunoto and her family have lived in and cared for her husband's brother's house, rent free. The small house is made of boards and has a rough ground floor. Light comes from candles, and they wash in well water. They do not have a proper lavatory and so use the general lavatory 100 meters away. The children use the veranda and then deposit the excrement in the ditch. They have a rubbish box, which they burn when it is full. The house contains a rack for plates, a trivet for cooking, a short table holding a stove, a bed, a wood rack with towels, a bed frame (without a mattress), a table for a lamp and radio, and a food cupboard. Sunoto either uses the trivet or a small stove for cooking. The kitchen equipment is very simple and includes one frying pan, two saucepans, and some plates and bowls. She has a small plastic feeding bottle, which her eldest son uses for drinking tea.

Both children were born at Dr. Kariadi Hospital in Semarang. The youngest received Lactona infant formula by bottle for the three days she was in the hospital. After that the baby received breastmilk only and no breastmilk substitutes. At seven days, Sunoto tried giving the baby mashed banana, but the baby would not eat it. At eight months, the baby was given soft-cooked rice, but again, she vomited, and so it was stopped. When the baby was one year, she was given mashed cassava cakes and she liked them very much. Eventually, the baby began to eat rice and the other family dishes. Sometimes the father brings them *tahu* (soybean cakes) from the factory where he works. Whenever she offered solids to her daughter, she rejected them, and Sunoto concluded that she did not like them and that they did not agree with her, and so she stopped offering them. Now at eighteen months, her daughter eats cassava cookies, bananas, and rice mixed with spinach and tahu.

She breastfeeds her baby whenever the baby cries and does not follow a schedule. She knows breastmilk is good and that it is better than canned milk. She eats lots of vegetables and drinks herbal tonics (*jamu*) to increase her breastmilk. When breastfeeding, she avoids eating fresh fish, red peppers, and young bean sprouts so that the breastmilk will not have a bad taste. She does not drink much water when breastfeeding. To wean her daughter, she gives water or tea to the baby continuously whenever the baby wants it. Sunoto has never had any problems with breastfeeding.

When she was pregnant, she avoided eating pineapples, cucumbers, bananas, and certain vegetables and drinking hot drinks and iced sweet drinks. After childbirth, she took a number of different tonic drinks and used a *pilis* (paste of herbs) on her head. When she was pregnant for the first time, her grandmother prepared a *upacara mitoni* ceremony in Surabaya, serving ritually correct foods to insure a successful delivery.

When her children get sick, Sunoto first takes them to the traditional midwife in the area for a traditional curing ceremony. After the ceremony, she gives them Bodrexin (aspirin), and if they still do not improve, she takes them to a local polyclinic.

In spite of difficult living conditions, Sunoto has the support of her husband and mother to see her through difficult times. Inevitable crises in her life are dealt with through traditional Javanese ceremonies.

Amporn. Amporn, an attractive, shy woman of twenty-seven, came to Bangkok from Ubonratchathani province in the Northeast of Thailand eight years ago. She married a young man from Cholburi province and settled into a small house in the Pasricharoen area of Dhonburi, Bangkok. The house, which is attached to neighboring houses, opens directly on to a narrow cement path leading to a popular indoor market.

Amporn used to work as a baby sitter in a Bangkok household. Before taking the job, she completed a short course on child care and received a certificate attesting to her training. Her husband is a serviceman in the Royal Thai Air Force and is stationed upcountry in Chiang Mai. He comes to visit every three weeks. When her children were born, she quit her job. But since she considers that the family income of 3000 baht (U.S. $150 per month) is inadequate, she is trying to go back to work.

Amporn has three children; the youngest son, who was born at Sirirat Hospital in Bangkok, was two months old when the ethnographers first met Amporn. This infant was never breastfed, although Amporn tried to nurse once in hospital on the day of the baby's birth. Lactogen was given by bottle at the hospital from the first day of birth. When the infant began having diarrhea at home, she stopped giving Lactogen. In all, the baby suffered from sixteen bouts of diarrhea in two months. Each time Amporn would change the brand of formula and search out new advice from health professionals. At first, she took the baby back to Sirirat Hospital and was told that the problem was not the infant formula but her preparation. She must not be sterilizing the bottle well enough. But for preparing the bottles she used boiled water and kept it in a thermos. Later, she took the baby to a local health clinic and was told to put salt in a bottle of Sprite and give this to the baby. This, too, was not effective. She was then advised to try the popular Bear Brand infant formula available in the local market. When the bouts of diarrhea continued, she took the baby to Children's Hospital and was told to buy Prosobee, a soy-based infant formula "prescribed for diarrhea." Throughout this trying time, she was constantly urged by her neighbors to try whatever they used to feed their infants. Her husband, on the other hand, could not understand why she did not breastfeed, since it would save them the money they were spending on infant formula, medicines, and clinic visits and might keep the baby healthy. But since her other children had been fed from birth with Lactogen, with no difficulty, she had anticipated no problems with her youngest child.

Although she has no relatives close by in Bangkok to give her advice and support, she goes regularly to Arunyaprathet to visit her two older children who are living in a village there until they reach school age. Like Sunoto, Amporn follows traditional practices, such as the ceremony of shaving the "fire" hair of the baby, and follows food prohibitions for lactating mothers, although she is not breastfeeding; that is, she avoided beef, sea fish, and sour foods for two months after childbirth. By the end of the study, Amporn was back to work as a baby sitter, taking her youngest infant, now recovered from the earlier bouts of diarrhea, with her to work.

Comparisons

Rosa, Grace, Sunoto, and Amporn have more in common than the fact that they all struggle to raise their children under difficult circumstances. They are all migrants from rural or urban communities, seeking a better life in Bogotá, Nairobi, Semarang, and Bangkok. While Amporn, Rosa, and Grace are dependent on their neighbors for advice and assistance, Sunoto is more influenced by her family than her neighbors. Amporn, Sunoto, and Rosa retain a stock of traditional knowledge about child rearing—both ritual and practical—to carry them through the traumas of raising children amidst urban poverty. Rosa, Grace, and Amporn all took positions as domestic maids in wealthier households. Ironically, the one mother who did not breastfeed, Amporn, holds a certificate in child care. Household composition may be a strong determinant of infant feeding patterns. But these variables are not simple to analyze. Relations with husbands or companions constantly change for many women. Sunoto has a stable marriage and the support and responsibilities of a resident husband. Amporn's husband visits from his military assignment, and Grace's husband returns to their rural homeland often. Rosa's companion left the union before the twins were born.

Not surprisingly, the four women fed their infants quite differently: Amporn bottle fed with different infant formulas and supplementary foods; Sunoto bottle fed with infant formula for three days in the hospital and then breastfed exclusively until the addition of supplementary foods at one year; Grace combined breastfeeding with infant formula, glucose water, and family porridge; and Rosa fed her twins with breastmilk, S-26, sugar water, and a variety of soup mixtures.

Community Contexts

Rosa, Grace, Sunoto, and Amporn are not representative of their communities or their cities in a statistical sense, but their lives reflect the complexities of life in poor, urban communities in third world countries. These communities in their respective cities structure many of the options women have for feeding their infants, primarily through food marketing and health care systems. In Singapore, in the 1930s, Williams actually blamed communities for allowing conditions to deteriorate: "And so a baby is murdered by a community that permits the mother to live under such conditions and to discontinue breastfeeding" (1986:68). The following sections place these households in their broader community and urban contexts.

Guacamayas in Bogotá. Rosa lives in Guacamayas, an area southeast of Bogotá containing about 100,000 inhabitants, mostly migrants who came to Bogotá within the past thirty years. The neighborhoods of Juan Rey, La Peninsula, Guacamayas, La Gloria, La Victoria, Altamira, and El Rodeo all are characterized by high growth rates and insufficient public services for electricity, water, sewage, and garbage collection. Although health care services are available, there are not enough to meet the demand, and the inhabitants make substantial use of the informal health services in the area. Mothers complained that they were not treated well in the health centers and that the hours and treatments were not suitable for their needs. Crowded and expensive health facilities encouraged mothers to use the drug stores and urban curers as providers of health services.

This is a low-income area with high unemployment and irregular work opportunities in the informal labor force. Many women in the area work in domestic service, in very small businesses, or at home. Emergency cash is obtained by pawning their few household objects.

These neighborhoods grew up as squatter settlements and are technically illegal. The ramshackle houses often shelter several families. Particularly in the rainy season the shacks are very difficult to reach. One family of thirteen living near Rosa erected their own shack of boards; it had a tin roof, no windows, and an earth floor measuring fourteen square meters.

The city of Bogotá differs substantially from Nairobi, Semarang, and Bangkok. Bogotá, which had a population of 21,000 in the nineteenth century, has now become the fifth largest city in Latin America, with a population of over four million. Around 1938, the Colombian population was about 70 percent rural and 30 percent urban. Political and economic changes in the country in the following decades, however, resulted in major shifts in the distribution of the population. The cities were forced to absorb large numbers of rural migrants, and by the mid-seventies 60 percent of the population resided in urban areas.

Bogotá grew so rapidly that the city was unable to meet the

growing demand for jobs or to provide the migrant population with adequate public services such as clean water, transportation, housing, and sewage disposal. The deteriorating conditions in the areas where migrants and low-income families live are reflected in the morbidity and mortality rates for children younger than five years of age. The community of Guacamayas exhibits many of the characteristics of these poverty belts around the periphery of Bogotá. Much of the migration is from urban and town areas, rather than directly from rural communities.

As in the poorest households in Bangkok, Nairobi, and Semarang, poor mothers in Bogotá spend much of their time struggling to obtain scarce and expensive resources. With endless lines for gas, water, and food, mothers have difficulty combining household and income-generating activities and creating conditions for keeping their children alive.

Kibera in Nairobi. West from Nairobi lies a housing development known as Kibera. Regular roads link the areas of middle-income apartments available for rent or purchase. Grace lives in the "villages," where semipermanent wattle and daub or wood huts, which have corrugated iron roofs, are serviced by narrow mud lanes. The "houses" are built in rows of eight to twelve single rooms of about ten square feet and rent for about U.S. $13.00 a month. Those with longer tenancy pay lower rents. A communal pit latrine and bathroom are located near these barrack-like structures.

In these squatter villages there is no electricity. Water taps, privately owned, are connected to the city water supply. Households purchase this water in four-gallon plastic containers for about five cents each and generally use about four containers a day. To save money, many women wash clothes in small "streams" running through the area. These "streams" are actually sewer outlets. Rubbish accumulates in front of the houses, along with feces of children who do not like to use the public latrines. Rubbish is burned or collected twice a week, and city authorities occasionally hire people to sweep the village clean, fearing a cholera outbreak.

The row houses of Kibera are not well served by transportation. Residents walk two to three kilometers to the main roads for bus service to Nairobi. Within the village area, a few tenants grow vegetables in open stretches of land between the housing developments and a few households illegally keep chickens and goats for food and emergency cash. Most food supplies are purchased from local kiosks. In the middle-income housing developments of Kibera there are modern shopping centers.

Kibera's location close to the major industrial area of Nairobi is beneficial for those fortunate enough to have regular jobs as unskilled laborers. Women in the villages of Kibera have few employment possibilities. A few obtain casual jobs as housemaids, seamstresses, or sell necessities like shoes or produce at small kiosks outside their homes. The largest government hospital is quite close to Kibera, and residents are also served by maternal and child health clinics. Although primary schools are available in Kibera, there are not enough places for all the local children.

Nairobi, Kenya's capital, grew up as an administrative center that serviced the needs of the British colonial administration. The city of over one million is undergoing rapid population increase, reflecting the 3.9 percent annual rate of population growth in the country itself—the highest rate of increase in the world. In 1975, Nairobi had 57 percent of all Kenya's manufacturing employment and two-thirds of its industrial plants. In 1979, the city contained about 5 percent of the national population (World Commission on Environment and Development 1987:238).

In the early days of colonial rule, the city was socially segregated, with areas designated for Asians, Europeans, and Africans. The African areas in particular suffered from inadequate housing, which lead to overcrowding and the development of illegal squatter settlements like Kibera. Encouraged by the colonial government, associations in Nairobi formed along ethnic lines. In addition, particular ethnic groups came to dominate certain occupations: Kamba in the Public Works Department, Luo as skilled aritsans, Kikuyu charcoal sellers from Nyeri, etc. (Furedi 1973:231). Kikuyu, the largest ethnic group in Kenya, accounted for over 40 percent of the population of Nairobi. In addition to ethnic associations, church membership is particularly important.

Nairobi is a city of rural migrants, mostly young males. In the early decades of the century, males migrated alone as casual laborers on short-term contracts. In the mid-seventies, less than 5 percent of adults had been born in the city, and few spend their entire adult lives there (Ross and Weisner 1977:363). Links between rural and urban households are exceptionally strong and sustained, even after urban migrants have become relatively successful. Women often work rural homesteads and join their husbands only in the slack agricultural season. In fact, women were not an important part of the labor force in Nairobi until after 1952. Until the mid-forties, most domestic jobs were closed to women (Furedi 1973:227).

Krobokan in Semarang. Located in the suburbs of west Semarang, this new urban residential area, covering more than 200 acres, has over 17,000 residents, including Sunoto and her family. The facilities were provided as part of a city development program and expanded through a Kampung Improvement Project in 1980. Roads are now paved with asphalt and equipped with electric lighting, and the ditches have been cleaned out. The suburban community, with its wider roads and larger yards, has a much more open and prosperous feel than inner-city communities. The homes are a combination of European-style brick housing and simple village-style housing of bamboo and wood.

Facilities within the community vary by family income. Piped water and electricity are available to those families who can afford them. However, around the railway tracks and by the river, sanitary conditions are particularly poor; in these areas the river is used for bathing and for toilet facilities. The Department of Public Works dumps garbage in the side streets near the river. The residents shop at nearby large markets, although the same items can also be purchased at local stores within the suburb. Public transportation to these larger markets is mainly by pedicab.

The area contains educated, middle-class families with a regular income, poorer families who work as daily laborers, and others who live as tenants, dependent on others. Poor women who are active participants in the PKK (family welfare association) make particular use of a revolving credit lottery. The PKK also assists with the preparation of traditional Javanese rites of passage to celebrate births, pregnancies, birthdays, and weddings. There are a number of religious organizations in the area, which include strict Islamic groups of men or women meeting for prayer and teaching.

Semarang, located on the north coast of Central Java, is the fifth largest city in Indonesia and the fourth most densely populated city in the nation. It has a long and complex history. Most reports suggest that Chinese traders settled in the area during the Ming dynasty in the 1400s. When the Dutch East India Company expanded its commerical activities in Java in the seventeenth century, a substantial group of Chinese merchants and traders was already there. In 1678, Semarang was turned over to the Dutch East India Company, which expanded the port facilities and built a fortress at the site. Around 1850, the central part of Semarang was designated as the Chinese quarter, and resident Chinese were required to live in this sector. As the city's population expanded and the Dutch residents left, residential segregation decreased, but the central commercial areas of the city are still predominately Chinese.

In 1976, Semarang expanded to include some of the surrounding rural subdistricts within its municipal boundaries. In spite of the attempts by city administrations to restrict the flow of rural migrants into Javanese cities, poor migrants continue to flock there looking for possible employment. Many of these people migrate only temporarily into Semarang and return to their rural families when they have earned some cash. These circular migrants, both men and women, often work as petty traders, supplying ready-to-eat food and drinks to all areas of the city. These food vendors provide snacks and infant foods such as porridges at very low cost. Constant travel for the purpose of work blurs the distinctions between rural and urban households.

Within the city of Semarang there is great intracultural diversity: Chinese merchant families, itinerant peddlers, strict Moslem civil servants, and prostitutes all may live in the same neighborhood. In attempting to understand the categories of people within the city, several distinctions are useful. First, among the category of Chinese, there is an important distinction between *totok* or China-born Chinese, and *peranakan,* Chinese born in Indonesia usually of Indonesian mothers. The latter do not usually speak Chinese, although they may have Chinese names. Second, Javanese themselves distinguish between: (1) *abangan* or *wong cilek* (small people), peasant farmers who practice a variety of syncretic Javanese rituals, most significantly the *slametan* or ritual feast; (2) *santri,* followers of strict Moslem practices, usually richer peasants and merchants; (3) and *prijaji,* the hereditary aristocracy perpetuating Hindu-Javanese court traditions, usually government workers or more educated upper middle class. These differences in religious practice are significant because they orient families and households around different key values.

Phasicharoen in Bangkok. Amporn's Bangkok home is in Phasicharoen, an old community that grew up around the commerical activities of the earliest Chinese settlers who grew betel nuts and the complexes of temples and palaces built by King Rama, the Sixth. Like other communities along the Chaophraya River's outlets, Phasicharoen was primarily accessible by canals and minor waterways. Currently, it is also easily accessible by roads and public transportation. The community is conveniently located near many health facilities such as Bangphai Hospital, Yawarak Hospital, Bangkok Metropolitan Health Station No. 33, Sirirat Hospital, and many private clinics and pharmacies.

The community has a central marketplace that serves local residents and those from adjacent areas. Two large markets play a dominant role in the daily life of the community by providing food and household necessities. Business and trading in the community, though not as active and busy as in the earlier decades, still adequately serve the needs of the community. Business activities here take place both inland and on the waterways. Fruits, vegetables, noodles, coffee, and soft drinks are sold by boat vendors. Restaurants, grocery stores, stationery stores and bookstores, hair stylists, tailors, and mobile food vendors all provide services and employment for local residents.

Bear Brand powdered milk is the only kind of powdered milk for infants sold in the local grocery stores. Other milk products include sweetened condensed milk of various brands, homogenized milk, and evaporated milk. Anyone who wishes to buy other brands of infant formula must go to the drugstore located right next to Chaorensri Market. There Nan, S-26, Lactogen, Bear Brand, and Meiji are sold. Other brands are available in larger department stores not too far from the community.

Although Phasicharoen as a whole is middle to lower income, there are also wealthier households in the community, descendants of those noble families associated with the old palace of the former queen of King Rama the Sixth. Poor households such as Amporn's live in rented two-story row houses in poor condition. These households are densely packed together, creating environmental and sanitation problems. Because these houses are rarely connected to water pipelines, water is stored in large jars. Toilet facilities are minimal. The poor make more use of canal water for bathing, washing, and cleaning.

Many residents of this community are government officials; others are in the armed forces. Laborers, shop owners, vendors, and drivers live side by side. Most women work close to home. Cottage industries are popular here because women can earn extra cash without leaving their children. These jobs include, for example, sewing bras, making umbrellas, working leather, and managing shops. Average income per month of those living in the community is somewhere around 4,000 baht (U.S. $200) per month. The average income of Bangkok households in 1982 was 4,231 baht per month (Xoomsai 1987:11).

Bangkok is a gigantic city of over five million people, spread over 1,537 square kilometers on both sides of the Chao Phya River. A primate city, which is over forty times larger than the next largest Thai city, Bangkok displays all the problems shared by other large Asian cities—pollution, overcrowding, traffic congestion, crime, prostitution, and unemployment. As a result of rapid population growth of the capital, and rising gas and food prices throughout the seventies, the cost of living for both urban elite and urban poor increased dramatically. In the early seventies, the inner core area of Bangkok, covering 21 square kilometers, had a population density of 39,000 inhabitants per square kilometer. This concentration of people and activities in the central core of the city has not diminished in the past decade. However, population has spread out to the suburban fringes as well.

As the center of the political, economic, religious, and cultural life of Thailand, Bangkok attracts temporary and permanent migrants from all parts of the country. The city sets the values and standards for the country, and migrants are prepared to endure difficult conditions in order to have access to the opportunities available—or presumed to be available—there for work, education, health, and recreation. Once migrants have arrived in the city, links with rural villages are maintained by visits from relatives seeking opportunities in the city and occasional visits upcountry for festivals and family crises.

The migrants survive and occasionally flourish because of the dualism of Bangkok's economy. Although most major domestic and foreign companies are located in Bangkok, they cannot employ everyone looking for work in industry and commerce. More significant for recent migrants is the large informal sector that provides a vast range of goods and services. The informal sector employs individuals—including children—who work irregular hours, negotiate prices, and produce goods for a small-scale bazaar-type economy.

About 10 percent of the Thai population can be identified as Chinese or Sino-Thai. Of these, over half live in urban centers. Thailand is often cited as a model of successful Chinese assimilation. In the nineteenth century, male children of Thai-Chinese parents could be registered as Thai or Chinese, while female children were automatically Thai. Later, all children born in Thailand automatically became Thai citizens. Since Chinese formal education is no longer available, and Chinese immigration is all but ended, Sino-Thai assimilation appears inevitable. The process is difficult to study because Sino-Thai take Thai names. By public consensus, certain neighborhoods are identified as Chinese, and within these many families can trace their descent to Chinese immigrants two or three generations back.

World System

Rosa, Grace, Sunoto, and Amporn, their children, and their households are located in very different kinds of urban communities, reflecting very different historical and cultural conditions. Although the women share the problems of living in poverty within poor, urban communities, neither they nor their communities are socially isolated or unaffected by broader social and economic pressures. Colombia, Kenya, Indonesia, and Thailand are part of the large, unified hierarchical system known as the world system. Rollwagon defines the world system as "a cultural system of elaborations and interpretations that structures the nature of the major economic transactions of the world and thereby influences the nature of the other functionally related cultural systems" (1980:375). The four countries are affected by many of the cultural processes common to the world system and are linked by many of the same institutions that crosscut national boundaries. Although the four countries in the infant feeding study appear to have little in common, they are all intricately connected with each other and with the world system. They cannot be considered simply as isolated cities or nations.

Infant feeding patterns are affected by the broad political and economic context of the world system. These processes include urbanization, colonialism and neocolonialism, industrialization, trade, capitalization of agriculture, international and national migration, and tourism. Historically, these processes are closely interconnected, as the industrialization of Europe is linked both to capitalism and colonialism. The raw materials, cheap labor, and large markets of the developing countries continue to attract neocolonial ventures. In Southeast Asia, for example, the new international division of labor encouraged the development of the American semiconductor industry. This industry, and the textile and garment industry, are known for their "superexploitation" of young women. In Thailand, the migration of young women from rural landless families to Bangkok was encouraged by the capitalization of agriculture and the demand for cash crops that began in the last century. Plantation agriculture in Kenya under colonial control first encouraged male migration and currently provides sporadic employment for rual and urban women around Nairobi. These four countries, all at various stages of development, share this feature in common: "they do not have external colonies to exploit and they are faced with pre-existing industrial states with the power and the will to intervene in their internal affairs" (Wallerstein 1974:280). Clearly, world systems operate to the benefit of some individuals, institutions, and countries and to the detriment of others.

Urbanization assumes different forms depending upon the historical, social, economic, and cultural contexts. In order to assess how the urban environment affects infant feeding patterns in each of the four cities studied, the cities must be placed in an even broader context. The cities differ in size, history, organization, and in their relations with the surrounding rural population. Three of the four cities display evidence of their colonial pasts—a distant past for Bogotá (Spanish) and a more recent past for Nairobi (British) and Semarang (Dutch). Bangkok is unique in its lack of colonial control. However, the city is strongly influenced by American, European, and Japanese interests.

The world system also produces institutions that cross national boundaries. The Roman Catholic Church, the World Bank, the World Health Organization, the Ford and Rockefeller foundations, and multinational food and pharmaceutical companies are all larger cultural systems that cross national boundaries. Elling adds to this list national bilateral aid programs, medical technology producers and supplies, polluting and exploiting industrial firms, agribusinesses, purveyors of chemical fertilizers and pesticides, and sellers of population control devices (1981:25).

The infant feeding project itself is an example of a supranational unit. By agreeing to participate in the study, each national team was affected by other supranational systems: the United States Agency for International Development (USAID), which sent out the original request for proposals, awarded the contract to the consortium, and funded the research; the multinational corporations such as Nestlé whose actions necessitated research and policy decisions regarding the marketing of breastmilk substitutes in the first place; and the United Nations organizations such as WHO and UNICEF, which placed the infant formula controversy on the agenda for international debate.

These three supranational systems, in addition to advocacy groups such as INFACT and IBFAN, which gradually became international organizations, had a substantial impact on the research process both in developing and developed countries. Thus, the very existence of the infant feeding project acknowledges some of the mechanisms drawing the four countries into the world system.

Consider the influence of the world system on the lives of the four women introduced earlier. Amporn's baby was born at a hospital with an internationally funded breastfeeding promotion program. But her continuous experimentation with different brands of infant formula was made possible by the competitive marketing strategies of European, American, and Japanese infant formula companies and their agents in Bangkok. Sunoto's infant was born in a western-style hospital in a health care system strongly influenced by decades of Dutch administration. Grace's regular attendance at a local Protestant church and the influence of the Roman Catholic Church on Rosa's self-identity are not isolated ethnographic observations but clues about broader processes and institutions affecting these women in their very different settings.

The influence of the world system on infant feeding practices in developing countries can be seen most clearly by focusing on the three topics developed in the following chapters—the empowerment of women, the medicalization of infant feeding, and the commoditization of food.

Women and the World System

The world system affects women directly and indirectly. Under British colonial rule, Kenyan women probably lost more rights and opportunities than women in the other countries. Yet Thai women may be undergoing more rapid transformations now under the combined pressures of assembly line factory work and sex-oriented international tourism.

In Thailand and Indonesia, women are preferred as workers in industries such as textiles and electronics because they are assumed to be docile and subordinate. Recently, strikes and efforts to unionize the textile industries in Thailand have disproved this assumption. In the eletronics industry, 85 percent of the workers are women (Mattelart 1983:111).

The shift of the American semiconductor industry to Southeast Asia occurred because the rising cost of production and organization of labor made capital accumulation more difficult. But in countries like Thailand and Indonesia, the presence of a low-cost, unorganized labor force—mostly women—made it possible to increase profits again. In the seventies, Indonesia and Thailand took over large-batch standardized low-grade production activities (Henderson 1986:101). Henderson points out that in 1980, foreign manufacturing rates were lowest in Southeast Asia, compared to American wages, with Indonesia and Thailand providing the lowest wages (1986:102).

In many industries in all four countries, women are hired on three- and six-month temporary contracts or on a daily basis so that they cannot claim benefits, particularly maternity leave, which are available only to permanent workers. Since these women lose their jobs when they are pregnant, there is little pressure for maternity leaves and lactation breaks from workers in these industries. Reform is complicated by the fact that "since multinational corporations locate in these communities principally because of the presence of cheap female labour, attempts to demand better wages, working conditions, job security, and advancement prospects often induce further capital flight" (Sen and Grown 1987:35).

Other supranational cultural systems may also influence women's self-image and ultimately have an impact on infant feeding decisions. Although religious ideology should not be mistaken for either beliefs or normative standards, ideas that women are impure, that breastfeeding is a women's duty, that maternal sacrifice is expected, or that standards of modesty preclude breastfeeding in public provide a context for women's decisions about infant feeding. Protestant churches, Roman Catholicism, and Islamic reform groups—all supranational cultural systems—link individual women like Rosa and Grace to broad systems of interpretation of gender-appropriate behavior that originate far from the communities in which these women reside.

Perhaps a more potent source of new gender images comes from the growth of international tourism, particularly in Bangkok, and to a lesser extent, Nairobi—both important centers for the tourist industry. Tourism provides service sector jobs in Bangkok and communicates powerful images of modern consumption patterns. It accentuates the inequalities between individuals and nations. For example, while Grace pays for each plastic container of water, multinational hotels in downtown Nairobi feature flowing water fountains and full swimming pools—a clear example of the differential impact of the world system in the same city.

It is tempting to blame the tourist industry in Thailand for creating the image of women as sex objects. In 1980, the total number of prostitutes in Thailand was estimated at between 500,000 and 700,000 (Sukanya 1981:5). Both the "push" of landlessness due to the capitalization of agriculture and the "pull" of relatively highly paid service sector employment encouraged the migration of young women to Bangkok. In all probability, the combination of poverty, women's increasing economic dependence on men, and the commoditization of sex all encouraged the growth of prostitution in Thailand. The expanding international tourist trade benefited from and sped up these processes considerably. Because of these and other other linkages to the world system, the empowerment of women is critical to understanding changing practices in infant feeding.

Medicalization and the World System

The spread of western biomedicine and hospital-based systems of health care throughout the world provide clear examples of the influence of the world system on the lives of individual women. Even in Semarang where 44 percent of the sample mothers gave birth at home, a poor woman like Sunoto may give birth in a large western-style hospital where infant formula is routinely given to all newborns for the duration of their stay in the hospital. Grace and Amporn both submit to the authority of their doctors without question. Other mothers "shopped around" and used health professionals as sources of information and free samples. Although there are great cultural differences in the plural health system operating in the four countries, the dominant hospital-based clinical model, derived from western practice, influenced changes in infant feeding practices in the four cities.

A number of supranational cultural systems assist in the

transmission of western biomedical models, among them, international organizations such as the World Health Organization (WHO), UNICEF, international medical associations, and the European, Japanese, and North American food and pharmaceutical companies. Mothers often differentiated between a wide range of specific brands of medicines or infant foods that they favored for their children. The development and direction of the Thai health delivery system was strongly influenced by the Rockefeller Foundation, which funded the medical education system in a number of countries. These supranational cultural systems continue to exert influence through training programs, consultancies, collaborative research, and regional seminars (see Higginbotham 1984). These and other linkages to the world system encouraged the medicalization of infant feeding, a topic explored in Chapter Four.

Commoditization of Food and the World System

Rosa, Grace, Sunoto, and Amporn participate most directly in the world system as consumers of products like Lactogen, Similac, Cerelac, Nestum, Nescafe instant coffee, Ovaltine, Coca-Cola, Ribena fruit syrup, Maggi soups, and Palmolive soaps, to name but a few products familiar to North American consumers. Companies like Unilever and Nestlé are key institutions in the definition of new food consumption patterns. The sight of a McDonald's in a major Thai shopping area is a reminder of the impact of the world system on even such culturally defined domains as meal patterns. Similarly, the great proliferation of different brands of breastmilk substitutes and weaning foods promoted by multinational food and drug companies is what the breast-bottle controversy is all about.

Mattelart identifies another transnational institution in addition to food companies implicated in these changes in patterns of consumption—the transnational advertising companies such as J. Walter Thompson, McCann-Erikson Worldwide, and Batten, Barton, Durstine and Osborne, or their subsidiaries (1983:52). Women, as specialists in consumption, have advertising directed to them or are featured as sex objects to encourage consumption (Mies 1986:120).

The world system assigns values to activities and products, including activities like breastfeeding and products like Lactogen. These values are easily transmitted to women like Rosa, Grace, Sunoto, or Amporn through the numerous supranational cultural systems affecting their lives. By documenting these connections, we run the risk of painting a very deterministic picture of living environments bombarded by western products, institutions, and messages. Certainly, these four women have some choices as to how they participate in the world system, but they cannot choose not to participate in it. Thus, in each city, even a confident and determined breastfeeding mother is surrounded by a competitive marketing and distribution system for breastmilk substitutes and a hospital and clinic system geared to the use of infant formula and bottle feeding.

Yet there is even more potential for distortion by picturing these women and their communities as part of isolated urban systems unconnected to each other and to the political and economic processes shaping the world system. These women are not part of static systems, even if the balance of power always appears to swing toward wealthier and more powerful individuals, institutions, and nations. Power can be redistributed throughout the world system, permitting subtle shifts in the orientation of key institutions and empowering new groups. In the seventies, new groups have gained influence in supranational arenas. Of particular importance to the infant formula controversy has been the strengthening of women's organizations and the coalitions representing consumer interests. Chetley and others have noted the rare instance of grass-roots organizations like INFACT and IBFAN gaining significant influence in institutions like WHO.

We cannot hope to examine the world system in its entirety, nor even its impact in the four countries involved in the infant feeding project in a single book. However, we can focus on processes that help explain changes in infant feeding practices. The most significant contexts for understanding both changing infant feeding patterns and the infant formula controversy are elaborated in the following three chapters on the empowerment of women, the medicalization of infant feeding, and the commoditization of food.

CHAPTER THREE

Infant Feeding and the Empowerment of Women

INFANT FEEDING, AND THE DECISIONS regarding breastfeeding and bottle feeding, are generally acknowledged to be women's issues. But this does not mean that infant feeding has been the subject of feminist analysis. Breastfeeding, and by extension the options for artificial feeding, should be and can be a paradigmatic feminist issue for significant feminist reasons. But lactation seems to have moved out of the consciousness of western women. It is not a central concern of women's health clinics or reproductive rights groups, nor is it something likely to be brought up in meetings on women's pay equity. It is surprisingly absent from contemporary feminist thought—much as if women no longer had breasts, or considered them merely as optional equipment. Other processes such as menstruation have not been similarly submerged and are part of the dominant feminist discourse about women's bodies. This chapter suggests how lactation became a submerged discourse and why it must be redefined and reinterpreted from a feminist perspective. We need to consider infant feeding and the breast-bottle controversy in the context of the empowerment of women, demonstrating first why this is a feminist issue and then reviewing some alternate paradigms used to interpret women's issues in the west. The complexities of the issue explain the lack of a single consistent feminist position on the controversy. However, if this argument reveals how the empowerment of women is linked to infant feeding decisions, then there are program and policy implications regarding infant feeding that follow from these observations.

INFANT FEEDING AS A FEMINIST ISSUE

Infant feeding, because it requires a decision on the part of women about breastfeeding, is a feminist issue. Feminism is defined here as a theory that analyzes and explains the causes of women's oppression and actively seeks the "eradication of gender subordination and of other forms of social and economic oppression based on nation, class, or ethnicity" (Sen and Grown 1987:18). The breast-bottle controversy is a feminist issue for both theoretical and practical reasons. Theoretically, the controversy helps us think through some of the most difficult dilemmas in feminist thought and action—the sexual division of labor and the fit between women's productive and reproductive activities. At the same time, it provides a focus for forming potential alliances between groups with very different agendas and philosophies. It is, then, an ideal issue for exploring the relation between theory and action.

The capacity to nurture infants and others, and to make things grow, is the basis of women's social production; it is basic to women's physiological and psychological well-being, self-esteem, and economic self-reliance. Conditions conducive to successful nurturing, including breastfeeding, are conditions that reduce gender subordination generally by contradicting negative images of women as sex objects, consumers, housewives, invalids, and welfare recipients. Conditions conducive to successful breastfeeding are also beneficial to women who do not bear children or who never breastfeed. More important, women, whether they breastfeed or not, are still affected by the forces promoting infant formula use and impeding breastfeeding—particularly the profit motives of multinational food and drug corporations.

Although there are many different ways to interpret breastfeeding from a feminist perspective, the following six reasons provide important directions for further feminist analysis. In brief, breastfeeding is a feminist issue because it encourages women's self-reliance, confirms a woman's power to control her own body, challenges models of women as consumers and sex objects, requires a new interpretation of women's work, and encourages solidarity among women.

1. Breastfeeding requires structural changes in society to improve the position and condition of women. Women need the opportunity to rest after childbirth, to have their basic needs met by others when they are most vulnerable, and to have a supportive person to assist with breastfeeding management and care for the newborn (see Raphael 1976). Since the nutrient requirements of lactating women are higher per unit weight than those of adult men, priority must be given to lactating women in the distribution of food. In some societies, lactating women may not receive enough food and nutrients to maintain sufficient milk production to ensure optimal infant growth. Breastfeeding focuses attention on the need to redress inequalities in the distribution of food and other resources.

Breastfeeding encourages women's self-reliance by increasing their confidence in their ability to meet the needs of their infants. Past research has shown that successful breastfeeding requires women to have confidence in themselves and enough self-esteem to protect (or in some contexts demand) their rights to breastfeed. In North America, Brack (1979) has shown that the more control women have over their own lives, the more likely they are to breastfeed their infants. She argues that breastfeeding decreases when women's social power decreases relative to that of men in their own groups. While a husband's attitude may be important, women with most control over their lives may be able to ignore negative attitudes that husbands might have toward breastfeeding better than women whose lives are more directly controlled by men. Women with a positive self-image may be less likely to assume that they do not have enough breastmilk or that their breastmilk is of poor quality.

An issue paper, *Women and Health,* lists what needs to be done to improve the health of women and children: the reduction of women's workloads, increased time for self-development and for health activities, an increase in women's income and education, and a general improvement in women's status (World Federation of Public Health Associations 1986:60). The links between breastfeeeding and the position of women have been made most clearly by Marie Savané: "The status of the breastfeeding mother is the central question in the debate . . . the improvement of women's social and economic status is basic to any change of attitude towards breast-feeding" (1980:82, 87). Successful breastfeeding, then, requires that the position and condition of women be improved, and that maternal health be made a household, community, and national priority.

2. Breastfeeding confirms a woman's power to control her own body and challenges medical hegemony. Successful breastfeeding reduces women's dependency on medical professions and discourages the further medicalization of infant feeding.

The knowledge mothers and midwives have about infant care and feeding increases in value.

When breastfeeding is seen as a feminist issue, the social and physical costs of breastfeeding are more carefully calculated. The costs include time and nutrients. This calculation accepts the idea that women's bodies are finite and cannot be overburdened without causing suffering and loss of their productive capacities. When women's systems are overburdened, maternal depletion would not be cited as a reason for increasing infant formula sales, but of increasing supports for breastfeeding mothers in the form of food and health care.

Part of a woman's power to control her own body concerns contraception. In spite of the spacing effects of lactation amenorrhea, breastfeeding women seek safe contraception, and they are particularly concerned to find contraceptives that do not affect the quality or quantity of their breastmilk. High-dose hormonal birth control pills may decrease milk production. Although contraception can be empowering for women, the search for safe contraception can be complicated by the fact that "many international pharmaceutical companies treat Third World women as guinea pigs for new methods; chemicals such as Depo-Provera (which is banned in most advanced industrial countries as dangerous to health) are widely dispensed to Third World women, often with the knowledge and participation of international agencies" (Sen and Grown 1987:48).

There is an assumption underlying research on women and health issues that as the position of women improves, so does the health, nutritional status, and general well-being of their children. In fact, the concept of maternal and child health developed from the recognition that the health of the mother and the health of the child influence each other (Whitbeck 1984:78). As women gain control of their own bodies and take more responsibility for their own health, they will be in a better position to care for their children.

3. Breastfeeding challenges the predominant model of women as consumer. The decision not to spend cash on breastmilk substitutes is a rejection of a consumption pattern forcing women to rely on delocalized, industrially produced foods. As purchasers of infant formula—an expensive product that is beyond the financial means of poor women in both developed and developing countries—women succumb to the dominant ideology devaluing breastfeeding and breastmilk. Women then seek commercial solutions to infant feeding, much as they reject other homemade foods and replace them with factory-made products. The need for constant expansion of commercial markets for these products fuels the advertising campaigns directed to women as consumers. For, as Mies asks, "Where would the national and multinational corporations sell their cosmetics, detergents, soaps, synthetic fibres, plastics, fast food, baby food, milk-powder, pills, etc., if middle-class women would not provide the market" (1986:207)? The desire to accumulate consumer goods to solve immediate household problems such as infant feeding, and to acquire goods as status symbols, is part of the process of modernization. But it is not without costs to women.

The pressure to buy is partly accomplished through advertising directed to women or using women as sex symbols. Even in China, the image of woman as "model worker" has been replaced by "woman the consumer"—of cosmetics, televisions, washing machines, etc.—sold through an image of a new Chinese woman curling her hair and wearing makeup (Mies 1986:207). Mies argues that mobilizing women to fulfill their duty as consumers has become one of the main strategies of capital in the industrialized countries (1986:125).

4. Breastfeeding challenges views of the breast as primarily a sex object. What are the historical and social conditions that force women to become so alienated from their bodies that they devalue their special capabilities and accept male defini-

tions of their worth? How did breasts become defined as sex objects for male pleasure? How did breastfeeding become interpreted as animal-like, obscene behavior, and breastmilk, a dirty, valueless, and potentially dangerous substance? Although in order to answer these questions the specific historical circumstances need to be defined for different social groups, westernization and modernization are implicated in the changing social attitudes toward the body. These processes of change are reflected in developing countries when feeding bottles are preferred in public, when women's reasons for choosing bottle feeding include fears that breastfeeding will alter the shape of their breasts, or when bad breastmilk is blamed for causing infant sickness. The Jelliffes write: "Westernization is associated with a shift in emphasis from the breasts' nurturing function in infant feeding to a primary sex-aesthetic function as emphasized in clothing . . . , advertising, and such visual entertainments as films and television" (1978:225). This is particularly relevant when this "mammary gland fixation" (Latham 1975:iii) discourages women from breastfeeding in public places for fear their breasts will be exposed to view.

These fears are more than confirmed when North American women are arrested for breastfeeding in public or asked to leave these places. Reports of women arrested for indecent exposure while breastfeeding in parks or shopping malls have reached the status of urban myths. Even when reports of harassment are exaggerated, public response to the events is particularly revealing. Gaskin describes the "First Canadian Suck-In"—a 1981 response to the expulsion of a nursing mother from a shopping mall, in which fifty Toronto mothers nursed their babies in the same shopping mall the week following the expulsion (1987:189). Commented one male observer, "To me, its just like urinating or defecating in public" (Gaskin 1987:201). Miss Manners's etiquette book reinforces this interpretation of breastfeeding as analogous to excretion.

She writes, "Would you change the baby's diaper on the dining-room table while people are eating?" (Gaskin 1987:201) Not all etiquette books share Miss Manners's view. *Charlotte Ford's Book of Modern Manners* agrees that, "No one should have to eat in a bathroom" (1980:328). Ironically, these attitudes toward public breastfeeding in North America have further strengthened connections between breastfeeding and excretory functions. Many North American women have probably shared the experience of having to breastfeed their infants while sitting on the floor or on the toilet in public restrooms. As Gaskin writes: "It is strange indeed that countries which so pride themselves on their fastidiousness should make social rules which often force their most vulnerable members to eat in places designed for the excretory needs of the other members of the society" (1987:200).

The embarrassment women may feel at the possible exposure of part of a breast when breastfeeding and their fear that breastfeeding will deform breasts or make them sag unattractively are the result of interpreting breasts primarily as sex objects. These interpretations undermine a woman's sense of worth and devalue her productive potential, making it easier to sell her commercial solutions in the form of breastmilk substitutes.

It is rare that the degradation of women expressed through interpretations of breastfeeding as obscene can be linked to violence against women. Yet one man interviewed during the protest of breastfeeding mothers at the Toronto shopping mall remarked that breastfeeding was the cause of "all the rape" (Gaskin 1987:189). Such a perverted comment is only likely to occur in a community where breastfeeding is private, rare, and considered slightly obscene.

5. Breastfeeding requires a new definition of women's work—one that more realistically integrates women's productive and

reproductive activities. In the sexual division of labor, infant care usually falls to women. While feminists argue how to redistribute the work of infant care more equitably, the fact remains that it is women who have the capacity to provide food for their infants, ensuring women's self-reliance and their infants' survival for the first few months of life. Research on how women's work activities affect infant feeding choices usually analyzes the rates of initiation and duration of breastfeeding for women working at home and women formally employed, or women's strategies for integrating breastfeeding into their schedules (see Van Esterik and Griener 1981).

The four-country study demonstrates that work outside the home is not the primary determinant of duration of breastfeeding, although it is strongly implicated in the early initiation of bottle feeding. Conditions at work and distance from work are extremely important also. But this research direction avoids the necessity of rethinking the concept of work from a feminist perspective, a necessary step before we can address the complex problem of how women's productive and reproductive work is defined and integrated in different societies.

Mies argues that lactation should not simply be viewed as a physiological function: "It is one of the greatest obstacles to women's liberation, that is, humanization, that these activities are still interpreted as purely physiological functions . . ." (1986:54). By stressing that women's bodies were the first means of production—of children and food—Mies argues that women consciously appropriated their own bodily nature to give birth and produce milk, forming not only units of consumption but of production as well. If the work of lactation is valued as productive work, not the duty of a housewife, then conditions for its successful integration with other activities must be arranged. These include maternity leaves, access to infants during work hours, flexible working hours, safe working conditions, and a living wage. When women's productive and reproductive work are devalued, the activities of both become alienated from each other and harder to integrate. Thus, Mies argues that we need a new feminist definition of labor.

The feminist concept of labor rejects distinctions between socially necessary labor and leisure and uses a mother as a model of a worker. For mothers, work is always a burden and a source of enjoyment, self-fulfillment, and happiness because the goal of their labor is the direct production of life, not the production of things or wealth (Mies 1986:216–217). Breastfeeding needs to be reinterpreted from this perspective. Mies argues that a feminist concept of labor stresses the maintenance of work as a direct and sensual interaction with nature, organic matter, and living organisms without mediation of machines (1986:218). This applies directly to the work of infant care: while breastfeeding is a direct and sensual interaction with an infant, bottle feeding requires the mediation of technology and male-dominated (and defined) modes of production.

6. Breastfeeding encourages solidarity and cooperation among women at the household, community, national, and international level. At the household level, successful breastfeeding requires the assistance of women, kin, or friends, to provide support in the form of information on lactation management and help with household tasks. Although women may manage successfully without this direct support in a community where "everyone breastfeeds," it is likely that women's support is everywhere beneficial to breastfeeding and may provide a valued and sanctioned opportunity for women to meet on their own terms. Although the concept of the *doula,* the person who "mothers the mother," is important (see Raphael 1976), Steady warns us against transporting a concept important in the context of the nuclear family to third world countries with vastly different systems of social organization (Steady 1981). In some settings, these support networks may

need to be formalized into breastfeeding support groups in areas, such as urban centers, where these networks are not sufficient. For example, the Breastfeeding Information Group in Nairobi has been particularly successful not only in person-to-person counseling and support, but also in monitoring infant feeding practices in hospitals.

The breast-bottle controversy encouraged collective activist responses from women in the creation of breastfeeding support groups in different developing countries. In North America, women supported the Nestlé boycott and formed the basis of the volunteer networks of local INFACT groups in Canada and the United States. Women, motivated by philosophies from left to right, organized boycott activities, wrote letters, and signed petitions about the controversy.

Hallman explains the role of women in the Nestlé boycott:

> Part of the explanation lies in the abilities of women in industrialized countries to identify with women in the third world who were being victimized by the high-pressured promotional efforts of the multinationals. Many women in our countries have experienced similar kinds of pressure to formula-feed rather than breast-feed when they have had babies. . . . It appears that women . . . have committed more time over the years to development education concerns. When a specific opportunity arose to take action, they were prepared to move. (1985:61)

An examination of the pattern of donations to INFACT Canada from 1980 to 1983 clearly shows that while women gave more as individuals (267 female donors compared to 66 male donors), group donations came largely from religious groups. The women's groups donating regularly were not feminist groups (with the exception of a feminist bookstore) but again were religious: Anglican and Catholic sisters accounted for forty-five donations and women's church auxiliaries for fifty-eight donations.

Of those groups most actively involved in the Nestlé boycott in 1979, the American INFACT mailing list shows only one La Leche League group membership, one feminist women's health center, six unspecified women's groups, and six YWCA branches. Although many donations came from individuals without group affiliation, the vast majority of supporters came from church groups in general rather than women's groups or feminist groups.

The boycott brought together women with very different approaches to women's issues. But feminist goals, however envisioned, require a variety of core activities: political mobilization, legal changes, consciousness raising, and popular education to deal with women's issues as they emerge. What is needed are coalitions and alliances cutting across different women's organizations and approaches to build a broad-based movement (Sen and Grown 1987:87). The breast-bottle controversy mobilized women to join related consumer groups such as Health Action International (concerned with marketing pharmaceuticals) and Pesticide Action Network and to rediscover for themselves how women in developed and developing countries are linked together through the operation of institutions in the world system.

Women are easily divided into feminists and women who blame feminists for current social problems, such as the destruction of the family. This makes it particularly difficult to find common ground. A *Newsweek* article cites a letter that states the division in clear terms: "I do not consider all working women . . . to be child-neglecting, emasculating, selfish vipers. It would be nice if I in turn were not regarded as a mindless, cookie-baking, gingham-clad nitwit" (Will 1978:100).

When North American women are divided against one another, they are less likely to recognize connections between conditions in developed and developing countries. In the infant formula controversy, these interconnections are quite explicit.

An increase in the rate of breastfeeding and slower population growth in developed industrial countries forced infant formula manufacturers to actively seek new markets in developing countries. The overproduction of dairy products in Australia and Europe initiated the need to create demand for specialty milk products in India (Mies 1987:132) and Southeast Asia (Robinson 1986; Van Esterik 1980b). The exploitation of women in electronics and textile factories in Southeast Asia depends on North American women demanding and consuming large quantities of consumer goods. For women working in these factories, the purchase of low-cost infant formula allows "them" to work for low wages without maternity leaves, so that "we" can continue to purchase low-cost consumer goods. Coalitions between women in developed and developing countries on issues like the infant formula controversy represent potential opportunities for recognizing common structures oppressing women and for proposing common strategies to change the position and condition of women.

The Position and Condition of Women

I have argued that the breast-bottle controversy is fundamentally a feminist issue. For many poor women, however, the power to define issues and take action on probable causes of their everyday problems does not rest with them. Feminism's commitment to breaking down structures of gender subordination is particularly difficult to accomplish when "gender subordination is deeply ingrained in the consciousness of both men and women and is usually viewed as a natural corollary of the biological differences between them" (Mies 1987:26). In the next section, I will examine some of the broader forces influencing the position of women in Thailand, Indonesia, Kenya, and Colombia and how these forces affect the definition of women's issues.

In the last chapter, we located Rosa, Grace, Sunoto, and Amporn in their urban environments and saw how these environments were linked to the world system. Now let us risk a crude measure of how these women reflect the position of women in their respective societies. These generalizations are necessarily crude and may distort more than clarify the complexities of gender relations and power. However, the sketches may show some of the structural differences influencing the position of women in each society.

Amporn and Sunoto. When writing of Southeast Asia, authors have stressed the complementarity of male and female roles in this region and the lack of exaggerated opposition of male and female ideologies. Factors that have been proposed to account for the relatively high status of Southeast Asian women include the availability of new frontier land in areas of relatively low population density, the division of labor for wet rice agriculture, and the absence in the past of strong centralized states (Winzler 1982).

On the other hand, other studies have stressed both the exploitation of Southeast Asian women—through prostitution, domestic service, and factory employment—and the effect of development on women. In spite of evidence for the social structural and cultural historical indicators of gender equality, there is increasing awareness that changes occurring within Southeast Asian societies, often referred to as modernization and development, may not always benefit women (see Stoler 1977).

There is an assumption of competence surrounding Amporn and Thai women generally—a quality that is apparent in the lives of women with minimal resources as well as in the lives of politically and economically privileged women. In a study of prostitution in Bangkok, Pasuk identified the following features of Thai social structure as demonstrating the important structural role played by women in Thai society: uxorilocal residence with men marrying in, bilateral kinship, equal inheritance of family property among sons and daughters, the existence of female spirit cult groups, flexible division of labor between men's and women's work, and women's management of family finances (1980:7–9). Flexible division of labor combined with female control of family finances strengthen Thai women's participation in the public domain.

Thai women, both rural and urban, have a very high rate of participation in the labor force and Thailand is often cited as a country with one of the highest rates of female work participation in the world. It is an economic necessity for poor and middle-class Bangkok households to have two incomes to meet basic needs and compensate for the irregularity of incomes. For Thai women, much of their personal identity appears tied to their work. In a survey of 500 Bangkok women, 49 percent identified work as the most important factor in raising women's status (Thai Women's Professional Association 1976:40). The Hanks described the exhilaration that Thai urban women find when engaged in stimulating occupations beyond household duties (1963:448–449). However, female unemployment is high during the slack agricultural season and contributes to the increasing proportion of female migrants like Amporn in urban centers.

In addition to the important role women play in rice agriculture, they are increasingly committed to formal education, making up 48 percent of the enrollment in primary schools and 53 percent of enrollment in upper secondary schools (Bovornsiri 1982:72). While older women have a much higher illiteracy rate than older men, the gap is narrowing for younger women. In addition, women predominate in teacher training colleges and comprise 51 percent of the professorial staff at Thai universities.

Religious ideology contributes to the prevailing gender ideology by providing or reinforcing key images of masculinity and femininity. Theravada Buddhism, the religious affiliation of over 90 percent of Thai, does not elaborate sexual differentiation symbolically but rather stresses differentiation by age, morality, and ordination status. Although only males may be ordained as monks, there is growing pressure for female ordination and an increasing recognition of the importance of women as meditation teachers and lay supporters of Buddhism.

One consistent characteristic of female gender ideology associated with all cultural images of women in Buddhist Thailand is women as nurturers who support children, adults, and institutions with food. This powerful image stresses women's potency to feed—not merely their responsibility to feed—and is particularly significant because it may be a structural universal, important for understanding the construction of gender ideology generally (Van Esterik 1986b).

Amporn does not belong to any of the formal or informal women's groups in Bangkok. Women's groups in Thailand include formal bureaucracies such as the Women's Council of Thailand as well as the newer advocacy groups such as Friends of Women and the Women's Information Center. Their concerns cluster around specific exploitation of women related to contraception (Depo-Provera), prostitution, and sex-oriented tourism. When I discussed the infant formula controversy with the leader of one Thai women's group, she immediately saw the problem in terms of increasing the supply and lowering the price of infant formula in the country to assist working women. Even the consumers' groups have not been able to focus much attention on the issue in such a competitive market environment.

Sunoto, living in a city in Central Java, is part of a much more heterogeneous nation state than Amporn's Thailand. Because it is impossible to generalize across the many different island and ethnic populations, the following remarks only refer to the position of women in Java. In 1980, this area, which dominates the political and cultural life of the country, contained 61.9 percent of the total national population (Withington 1985:139).

As in Thailand, Javanese women are actively involved in rice production, although they appear to be losing certain opportunities because of the development of new agricultural technology. The flexible division of labor and women's management of financial resources strengthen their position in both household and community. Bilateral kinship with a bias toward uxorilocal residence favors the development of female work groups.

Gender ideology is strongly influenced by Islamic belief and practice, although both have been integrated with traditional beliefs and customary law (see Manderson 1983). An important concern is the purity of women: for example, when there is a blood discharge from the uterus, a woman is not allowed to fast, pray, or have sexual activity, for she is not *suci* or pure. A second dimension is *kodrat,* or women's natural inheritance or destiny. Her duty to husband and children is an important aspect of Javanese women's self-identity and cannot easily be ignored or jeopardized. Some Islamic sects segregate men and women and encourage practices that control the natural sensuality of women. The basic message of the Islamic reform movement is that "a woman's place is in the home" (Peacock 1978:48).

The Pancasila (the five principles of Indonesian nationhood) states the equality between men and women, technically ensuring the lack of discrimination against Indonesian women. Government policies stress that the primary responsibility of a woman is to her family, and women's programs seem to reflect this emphasis. An Indonesian feminist position appears to encourage policies that improve women's ability to care for their families. Women's issues are primarily focused on social welfare, including new marriage laws that would end child marriage, polygamy, arbitrary divorce, and unequal inheritance laws. Urban women have concerns about equal pay. It is interesting to note that as the government encourages family planning among Javanese women, some mothers' groups are demanding roads, water, and other services in return for their participation in government programs (Morgan 1984:315).

Sunoto recognized what other authors have confirmed about many women's groups in Java—that they are middle- and upper-class groups, offering only advice (and access to a rotating credit lottery) to the poor. Recall that Sunoto was too ashamed to join her local PKK (family welfare association) where she would have been instructed in proper infant feeding practices and given weaning recipes. These groups actively promote breastfeeding and provide educational material for women to follow concerning infant care. However, the groups have not been actively involved in the controversy and leave the problem of infant formula to the consumer groups.

Grace and Rosa. Grace is strongly oriented toward her rural home. Most Kenyan women live in the rural areas, practicing subsistence horticulture and petty trading. Town and urban living is less significant for many Kenyan women, who often provide the major support for their children by farming. In spite of the importance of Kenyan women in the food production system, women were generally excluded under the wage labor system of British colonial Kenya. As men worked on settler farms and plantations for wages, women became the principal food producers for their dependents. Under colonial conditions, men had access to money from cash crops, although the money was used to pay taxes and not always spent on food purchases for the family. Under British colonial rule, which lasted until 1963, the major ethnic groups—the Kikuyu, Luo, Luhya, Maasai—were resettled in designated reserves. Men had further opportunities for employment away from the reserves, often in distant cities like Nairobi.

Life in Nairobi in colonial and postcolonial Kenya remains particularly difficult for women like Grace who are seeking work or joining their husbands in the capital. Employment opportunities are few and consist mainly of domestic service in wealthy African, Asian, and European households, or informal petty trade in vegetables and other household necessities. Women's access to employment in the formal sector is limited, and they rarely occupy government positions.

In spite of their importance in the food production system, Kenyan women face many obstacles to equality. Since school fees beyond primary grades are a substantial burden for subsistence farmers, families select against girls in sending their children to school, with the result that females have only a 10 percent literacy rate (compared to 30 percent for males). The education gap is closing between males and females, but females have a higher dropout rate than males (Kettel 1986:10).

Kenyan women's identity is closely tied to their children. This is reflected in the low percentage of women between the ages of fifteen and forty-nine using contraception (Morgan 1984:392). Women's distrust of contraception contributes to Kenya's high and growing birth rate. This identification of Kenyan women as mothers is shared by men who fear that women who seek new role definitions will neglect their families. Men try to control women by appealing to their commitment to their childbearing and nurturing roles. Gender ideology in Kenya can best be understood by reference to the cultural values associated with the sex-gender systems of the different ethnic groups in the country. For example, Grace is Luo, and her experience of patriarchy is derived from living in a patrilineal society influenced by Christian missionizing. About half of Kenya's population identify themselves as Christian and about one-quarter as Moslem. The values concerning masculinity and feminity emerge from carefully separated male and female domains, both of which are controlled by men. Because men are presumed to be different from women, women like Grace seem to be very patient and careful with men, careful to avoid doing or saying anything that would expose men to public ridicule. This ideal of supporting and protecting male identity can be seen even under conditions of male neglect or abuse of women.

In spite of these obstacles, Kenyan women are actively involved in development projects that will benefit their communities rather than benefit women as a category. Government community development departments have supported locally organized women's groups that have sought to introduce new standards of health and nutrition. Over 600,000 Kenyan women are actively involved in local self-help groups (Kettel 1986:10). These groups participate in farming and livestock management projects, community development, handicraft production, and trade.

In addition to these self-help groups, Kenya has government-sponsored women's organizations such as Maendeleo ya Wanawake (Progress of Women) and the National Council of Women. As in Thailand and Indonesia, "the organizations are deeply divided between the elite women who run them, and the alienated local women whose interests are not served by them" (Stamp 1987:68). These women's organizations enthusiastically endorse breastfeeding promotion campaigns and breastfeeding support groups. According to one Kenyan group leader, the western view that bottles liberate women makes no sense. She explained to me, "Breastfeeding is a woman's God-given right, and if she is not able to breastfeed her own child, how could she be considered a competent woman?" To her, competence as a breastfeeding woman is a precondition for competence in other domains, such as managing a bank. Yet this attitude can be turned against women. Wipper cites Peter Omija who took women to task for failing to be good mothers:

> The first vital duty of a woman is to be a good, humble, nursing mother, and as such a woman has no time for politics. African women are poor nursing mothers. In Kenya, millions of children from the age of one week to 12 years suffer from malnutrition and as a result of this kwashiorkor is prevalent in this country; not because there is no one to prepare good, clean, well balanced diets in the homes. This is because women go into activities which are unnecessary, leaving children at home in a dirty mess and going hungry all day. (1972:344)

Rosa, whose home is in the squatter settlements surrounding Bogotá, lives in a much wealthier and more developed country than the other three women. It is also a country with a much larger concentration of people in urban centers. Nevertheless, poor women on the margins of prosperous cities face comparable problems due to the lack of adequate public services, housing, and transportation. Living conditions are particularly difficult for female migrants like Rosa who have recently arrived from other towns and cities in Columbia.

Gender ideology appears more directly related to religion than is the case in Kenya. Almost all (96 percent) the population is nominally Roman Catholic, and there is a pervasive recognition of patriarchal authority in most Colombian institutions, including the family. Gender ideology builds on the opposition of masculinity, developed in machismo values of virility and sexual aggression, and Marianismo, the elaboration of spiritual superiority of women and maternal sacrifice (see Browner and Lewin 1982). The bilateral kinship system does not particularly favor women, although legally women do retain control of property they bring to marriage. That is of little use to Rosa, however, who brought few resources to her union and relied on men to support her and her children. But her unreliable, unstable relationships left her particularly vulnerable.

Colombia recognizes both civil and religious marriage, and divorce is legal only for civil marriage. The literacy rate is high for both boys and girls, thanks to their equal participation in the education system.

Women like Rosa have only restricted access to employment. In Bogotá in 1980, women made up only 25 percent of the labor force; over 50 percent of employed women are in the service sector or working part time. While women in the formal sector are protected by maternity leaves and related legislation, poor women like Rosa have neither employment opportunities nor social services to rely on. Women's groups in Bogotá are generally professional or church related and are organized to perform voluntary services and dispense charity.

INFANT FEEDING AS A WOMEN'S ISSUE

In the previous sections, I have briefly sketched something about the position of women in Thailand, Indonesia, Kenya, and Colombia. Even if we could document all the indicators of the status of women widely cited in the literature—measures of political, legal, economic, educational, and family status—it would not be possible to give a single indicator of the position of women in these four countries. Nor is this a productive exercise, since we have no way of evaluating which of these domains is more important for ranking males and females within a given society, and no way of demonstrating how power is differentially exercised within these domains (see Van Esterik 1987:597). The sketches should, however, give some indication of the kinds of institutions that affect women's lives, and hence their infant feeding decisions. Research discourse continues to fuel the search for indicators of women's status and factors predicting women's infant feeding decisions. The factors most commonly cited—economic status, household composition, education, and formal employment—help explain some infant feeding patterns within a country but fail to predict overall breastfeeding rates between different countries.

In North America and Europe, wealthier and better educated women are more likely to breastfeed. But studies have shown that the duration of breastfeeding is usually shortest among well-educated professional women in developing countries (Hofvander 1979:69). The WHO collaborative study on breastfeeding showed that wealthier urban women initiate breastfeeding less often and breastfeed for a shorter duration of time than rural or urban poor women. The WHO study reported that of those wealthy women in the Philippines and Guatemala who ever breastfed, over 50 percent weaned their children by the second month of life (WHO 1981:33). In Thailand, it is wealthier and more educated urban women who are giving up breastfeeding first, regardless of work status (Knodel 1982:310). In our study, work away from home, high socioeconomic status, and being born in Bangkok are related to a shorter duration of breastfeeding and early introduction of bottle feeding. Similarly, educated, urban-born Kenyan women who gave birth in hospitals have a shorter duration of breastfeeding. Higher-income women were more likely to use bottles early. In Bogotá, work and higher socioeconomic status were associated with shorter duration of breastfeeding. In Semarang, Java, where women breastfed for the longest duration, increased family income and physician-attended birth lowered the probability of longer breastfeeding. Work outside the home was related to early bottle feeding (Winikoff, Latham, and Solimano 1983).

These results from the four-country study fit well with other studies of infant feeding trends. The research designs and results may differ, but they suggest a disturbing paradox.

Increased education, literacy, income-generating opportunities, and access to modern health care facilities are all acceptable and common goals for strengthening the position and condition of women in society. Yet they also appear to be related to the decrease in initiation and duration of breastfeeding in developing countries. Do these trends suggest that as the position of women improves, they can afford to bottle feed and choose to do so rather than breastfeed, or that they can better care for their infants by working and using the cash to buy quality food for their infants? These research results, if taken out of context, obscure the complex relation between breastfeeding and the empowerment of women and raise the specter of the inevitability of artificial feeding as the norm as the position and condition of women improve. Often a simple causal link is inferred here, and in the absence of either advocacy conviction or a broader analytical framework, the important questions cannot be raised, let alone answered. Raphael asks, "is it possible that as the developing world takes on western values, the trend to the bottle may be irresistible and even inevitable?" (1985:145). Without a feminist framework, we are left with studies that illustrate only short-term analyses (and often vested interests) when what is called for is a willingness to grapple with the contradictions emerging from different feminist perspectives.

ALTERNATIVE FEMINIST FRAMEWORKS

Feminist writers and groups in North America have been slow to define the breast-bottle controversy as a feminist issue. Although the National Organization of Women in the United States and the National Action Committee on the Status of

Women in Canada both endorsed the Nestlé boycott, they did not develop the feminist potential of the breast-bottle controversy. It was not a "cause" that lent itself to a single feminist perspective because women viewed the controversy—and infant feeding decisions—as intensely personal and emotionally loaded matters. Opinions about breastfeeding run the gamut from extreme conservatism to radical feminism, and each position can be defended by reference to a broad appeal to "what is best for women."

I have already argued that breastfeeding and the infant formula controversy are feminist issues. What is harder to explain is the emotional extremes and personal biases that emerged throughout the controversy and the lack of feminist commitment to and critique of the issue. Although there is agreement among feminists in identifying certain features of contemporary society as oppressive to women, feminists differ in how to explain and analyze these features. These values affect not only the explanation of issues, but even the description of "the facts." Jaggar attributes these disagreements to differences in values connected conceptually to differing views of human nature (1983:170). There are a variety of ways to categorize contemporary feminist theory. The classification Jaggar developed serves as a useful framework for analyzing the deep-seated contradictions in the assumptions and ideological forces women and men bring to the infant formula controversy. The most significant positions include those that might be characterized as the conservative, liberal, radical, and socialist feminist arguments.

Conservative Arguments

Western feminists reject a conservative position that denies the oppression of women and accepts the proposition that human nature is determined by innate biological differences between the sexes. However, elements of conservative logic pervade the discourse on breastfeeding and bottle feeding, often through the guise of a resurrected maternal or domestic feminism. Historical maternal feminism and its logical continuation in the seventies and eighties stress the intrinsic moral superiority of women and motherhood as a sacred trust. In an editorial on "Feminism and Motherhood," Stuart-Hagge interprets feminism as the need to pursue "self-actualization." She writes: "It is my belief that the woman who chooses to make motherhood her career exemplifies feminism in its most basic form. . . . Because a child's primal attachment is with the mother, and because only she can breastfeed . . . her time and commitment cannot be duplicated" (1981:3–4). The logic of maternal feminism affirms devalued and subordinated values: "We, like the maternal feminists of the past, value many traits traditionally associated with the domestic sphere: nurturance, compassion, co-operation and interdependence" (Prentice and Pierson 1982:108).

But feminist rhetoric, and particularly the logic of maternal feminism, is also used by conservative, antifeminist groups to preserve the status quo. New conservative feminism, growing in popularity and support in North America, defines itself as pro-family, celebrating feminine and nurturant qualities associated with mothering (Stacey 1983). The new conservatives claim that the feminist movement denigrates housewives and mothers and seeks to destroy the family. Conservative reasoning underlies some infant feeding policies and programs, even when couched in more widely acceptable feminist rhetoric. What are the concepts that keep the conservative position represented in the infant feeding controversy?

Conservative messages stem partly from the facts of women's reproductive capacity. Lactation as part of our mammalian heritage is suppressed only with difficulty (and some discomfort) through medical intervention such as pills or injections to suppress lactation. Breastfeeding is thus seen as the natural continuation of pregnancy and birth. Conservatives make much of the "naturalness" of breastfeeding, which increases the confusion of mothers who encounter breastfeeding problems. In some parts of the world, "natural" breastfeeding involves nearly continuous body contact between mothers and infants, as if the infant is still a part of the mother and symbiotically identified with her (Simpson 1980:17–18).

Rossi's arguments that "the interconnections between sexuality and maternalism make good evolutionary sense" angered feminists (Eisenstein 1983:70), who interpreted her argument on biosocial parenting as reinforcing old conservative stereotypes based on biological determinism. She argued that feminists had gone too far in rejecting women's nurturing role: "The full weight of Western history has inserted a wedge between sex and maternalism so successfully that women themselves and the scientists who have studied their bodies have seldom seen the intimate connection between them" (1977:17). In her defense, Rossi argues that we need to know more than we do about bodily processes, including lactation.

According to conservative logic, women are totally fulfilled only through pregnancy, birth, and lactation. It is but a small step to assume that it is women's primary duty to stay home and care for children, and if she has difficulty with or rejects this role, "she might ask herself if there isn't something wrong with her attitude if she regularly finds the duties of motherhood unpleasant" (Blackman 1981:283). These elements are reflected in one of the best and most widely used manuals on breastfeeding, *The Womanly Art of Breastfeeding,* written and published by the La Leche League. Although first written in the 1950s, its subsequent revisions continue to make value judgments concerning women's duties and the naturalness of breastfeeding: "The nursing mother, of necessity, stays at home; the father of necessity, will go out and make a living. The wifely duties will consist of baby and child care, cooking, washing, ironing, and the many tasks usually associated with homemaking" (La Leche League 1976:115).

Conservative themes are also reflected in literature and programs that stress the need for modesty by keeping the breasts covered while breastfeeding; that give assurances that breastfeeding will not endanger the sexual appeal of the breasts by making them sag, or in fact, make reference to the fact that men may be even more attracted to the enlarged breasts of a lactating mother; and that express concern that mothers obtain the approval and support of their husbands for breastfeeding. Although these points in themselves may be practical suggestions for some women in some societies, it is important to recognize the conservative assumptions underlying them in order to more fully understand the emotional fervor of the infant formula controversy.

Finally, conservative reasoning underlies the shift in emphasis from mother's rights to infant's rights. In a radical feminist discussion of breastfeeding, Evans notes that "many of the books about breastfeeding that are available now are written by people who believe that a baby has a right to its mother's milk, no matter what her feelings on the alternatives are . . . if she shows revulsion at the idea of breastfeeding, she's told she's being selfish and lazy" (1980:51). The La Leche League and various movements that support more natural childbirth and mothering can become oppressive as they develop ideals and standards against which mothers judge themselves and are judged.

Conservative views of modesty and sexuality may underlie women's decisions to bottle feed, while equally conservative views of breastfeeding as women's natural heritage and duty may underlie women's decisions to breastfeed. More significantly, because there is not an adequate feminist analysis of the contradictions posed by breastfeeding, women are more likely receiving a double message:

> A woman lactates: She understands that she should be proud to fulfill her destiny in this way. She is told that this is the best way to nourish her baby, no milk is comparable to human milk. She is taught to do it discreetly though, so as not to offend passers-by when acting out her proud destiny. She gets to understand that after having fulfilled her destiny, the altered shape of her breasts may render her less sexually attractive. (Helsing 1979:72)

Liberal Arguments

The early second-wave feminists who led the liberation movement of the sixties and seventies wanted to see opportunities increased for women in order for them to "catch up" with men and participate more fully in the mainstream of modern society. Their efforts to remove sexual discrimination included improving educational opportunities and legal rights for women and lobbying for equal pay for equal work. Liberal feminists, however, are less concerned with critiquing either conservative or radical feminist positions than with ensuring that women have full access to the benefits of western society. They do not question the causes of inequalities in western society, but work to remove gender inequalities to ensure that women will be more central to the activities valued in mainstream North American society. Liberals phrase women's liberation in terms of individual rights—rights to choose abortion, rights for children—that are often defined legally. They generally share with more radical feminists the desire to challenge the sexual division of labor so that child care comes to be shared more equitably between men and women.

From a liberal perspective, breastfeeding might well be viewed as restrictive and unappealing, tying an otherwise emancipated career woman to the restrictive roles of wife and mother. For these women, infant formula and bottle feeding are part of the technological solution to the problem of making their reproductive and productive lives more compatible. In their view, bottle feeding, child care centers, and maternity leaves allow women to compete more equitably with men. This position is reflected in a recent study of "post-liberated" American women. There is only one reference to breastfeeding in the chapter on families of the future:

> Until modern technology provided us with infant formula, we women didn't have much choice about who was to spend the most time with an infant. (I know breast-feeding is going through a popular revival among educated women today, but several generations of Americans grew up hardy and healthy on formula. Women who don't prefer or can't breast-feed shouldn't feel guilty about it.) (Duley 1986:151)

North American women who choose to breastfeed might well recognize existing discrimination against lactating mothers, object to the lack of facilities for nursing mothers to feed in comfort and privacy in the workplace or in other public locations, and argue for more extended maternity leave with no subsequent loss of seniority. However, liberal apologists may also oppose protective legislation for women on the grounds that it is a form of discrimination and may encourage employers to preferentially hire men. Other liberal arguments allow for legal reforms that compensate for biologically caused handicaps (Jaggar 1983:181).

It is the liberal position that is most compatible with the promotional efforts of infant formula companies in the west. Humanized infant formula, developed by the 1920s, did not become popular in North America on a large scale until World War II, when it freed more women to work full time for the war effort. Bottle feeding with new "improved" varieties of infant formula offered "liberation in a can" for working women. This is the argument that the infant formula companies present in their public relations efforts, including widely distributed movies

(Nestlé, *Infant Feeding: A Shared Responsibility;* Ross Laboratories, *Mothers in Conflict, Children in Need*). It is therefore ironic that at the WHO/UNICEF meetings in October of 1979, the working group studying ways to improve the health and social status of women in relation to infant and young child feeding had no industry representatives. Fourteen industry representatives attended the working group on the marketing and distribution of infant formula and weaning foods, a topic closer to their interests (Chetley 1986:66). Helsing points out that this misunderstanding of liberation led many feminists to reject one dispensable part of reproduction, lactation (1979:72).

Liberal positions generally ignore the deep contradictions between ideas of individual choice and the assumptions guiding key commercial and political institutions in North American society. These unresolved conflicts surfaced clearly in the infant feeding controversy. As with conservative positions, liberal voices were raised to defend both breastfeeding and bottle feeding, but always in support of the right of the individual mother to choose for herself.

Radical Feminist Arguments

A radical feminist position assumes that the oppression of women in all societies—socialist and capitalist—originates from their reproductive functions, which force them to become dependent on men. For some radical feminists, their political position requires them to separate themselves entirely from men by becoming lesbian. Radical feminists assume the existence of universal patriarchy and use the most powerful rhetoric and ideology to fight it. Political lesbianism is partly an attempt to create a nonsexist environment for women—a "womanspace" where the symbols and constraints of patriarchy are removed. It is the radical feminists who have made the most visible attacks on symbols of patriarchy such as pornography, rape, and sex-oriented tourism.

Radical feminists seek the fundamental restructuring of gender roles to allow both men and women to develop their full potential, freed of restrictive ideologies and practices. The flexibility they envision would include first, the right for women to choose whether they want to have children and second, if they do have children, the right to have more control over the total process of pregnancy, childbirth, and lactation. Radical feminists informed the Women's Health and the Reproductive Rights movements. A key issue for them is women's loss of control over their own bodies in the form of anesthetized, uninformed birth and other procedures that make it more difficult to establish lactation in the hospital. These procedures include binding the breasts, using drying substances to clean nipples, and the use of pills or injections to dry up the milk supply. This amounts to a "functional castration" of women who have "acquiesced to a combination of forces, medical and cultural, which have eventuated in the use of the breast as the primary sex symbol and yardstick of feminine desirability, divorced from its nurturing function" (Weichert 1975:987). Weichert makes a further analogy with artificial insemination as a routine medical procedure. "Would anybody suggest, seriously, that males abstain from intercourse, bind themselves, take drugs to relieve congestion, or be mechanically relieved routinely, and that it would be as good?" (1975:987). As feminists argued about *Our Bodies, Ourselves,* they reclaimed ownership and control over their bodies, allowing each woman to "experience her breasts in a new perspective; not as playthings . . . but as an erogenous zone where pleasure and function are inextricably intertwined" (Bloom 1981:262).

Yet radical feminist assumptions have also been used to support the position that breastfeeding and infant feeding methods are issues that simply are not on the agenda for political action. If motherhood is the basis of women's oppression, then lactation, too, is a part of the reproductive system oppressing women. But radical feminism produces contradictory arguments about motherhood. These women fight for the right to refuse motherhood while at the same time exploring the potential for lesbian mothers to experience pregnancy and lactation (through technological innovations such as artificial insemination) and embracing the concept of motherhood as the inspiration for feminist values and activities such as mother-goddess rituals. They have been criticized by socialist feminists for placing too much emphasis on sexual politics and viewing women "as vaginas and wombs on legs" (Jagger 1983:292–293). Their ahistorical and ethnocentric assumptions about universal patriarchy as the basis for the universal oppression of women make it difficult to apply western radical feminism to the analysis of women's issues in third world countries, although their passion inspired many international women's groups.

Socialist Feminist Arguments

Unlike radical feminists, who see the oppression of women as the primary form of oppression in all societies, socialist feminists consider gender discrimination to be inseparable from class discrimination. But unlike Marxist feminists, who assume women will be liberated when class oppression ends, socialist feminists combine political economy arguments with gender analysis (see Stamp 1988). This perspective encourages a broader examination of institutions in class societies that oppress women and a more cultural relativistic examination of the experiences of different groups of women in order to observe the interaction of class and gender relations in specific historical and cultural contexts and how they reinforce each other. This makes socialist feminist arguments more useful for application in third world societies than radical feminist arguments.

Socialist feminist positions on the infant feeding controversy would probably place the conflict squarely in the capitalist expansion of market forces into third world countries rather than in the context of sexual politics or the personal decisions of individual mothers. However, breastfeeding is not included as part of socialist feminists' view of reproductive freedom (Jaggar 1983:318). The transformation of social conditions that socialist feminists envision would generally be beneficial to breastfeeding, even though this issue is not defined as a primary concern. The development of self-help clinics for women, the increasing pressure for the use of midwives, and the increasing opportunities for informed, prepared natural childbirths in North America assist breastfeeding since these conditions enable women to exercise more control over their bodies and lives. The broader perspective of socialist feminism encourages examination of the way society and its institutions influence physiological processes like menstruation, menopause, childbirth, and lactation. Socialist feminist critiques of contemporary society point up the need for far-reaching social changes that would be beneficial to women, children, and men, as well as breastfeeding mothers in North America. These include maternity and paternity leaves, day care, nursing breaks, more flexible working hours, and other social policies women's groups have been fighting for (Richardson 1975).

Helsing locates the origin of the oppression of women in industrial capitalism, which forced women to compete with men without adjustments to meet the special requirements of women (1979:72). This argument, combined with the devaluation of women's productive and reproductive work under industrial capitalism, is the current direction of socialist feminist analysis. Eisenstein sees new feminist theory and practice emerging out of the recognition of gender as a significant political category, the retreat from false universalism, sensitivity to the diversity of women's experiences and needs, and linkages with broader justice issues (1983:141). This places socialist feminism in the best position to forge alliances with a broad range of women's groups and create a new integrative feminist framework.

Contradictions, Coalitions, and Backlash

The contradictory frameworks partly explain the emotional fervor and absence of a single feminist stance on the breast-bottle controversy. In fact, there are few informed feminist critiques on the controversy, although it is a powerful entree into a number of related women's concerns such as abortion rights, child care, and maternity benefits. Perhaps more significant are the coalitions that developed between wildly divergent ideologies. What ideological forces could align conservative and radical feminist positions on the "naturalness" of breastfeeding? The use of "natural" in the discourses on breastfeeding has distinctive meanings, depending on the context. The metaphor says very different things to very different women. Natural breastfeeding from a conservative perspective is based on the biological propensity for women to nurture children and others. Breastfeeding, to conservatives, is women's "natural" duty, along with other wifely duties such as child care, cooking, washing, and ironing. Natural breastfeeding from a radical feminist perspective is one of a series of changes that gives women more control over their reproductive processes and fits with natural childbirth and women's self-help clinics. Jaggar points out the irony of the radical feminist insistence on the political significance of reproductive biology, which challenges traditional conceptions of the "natural" basis of human life, while at the same time many radical feminists continue to treat reproductive biology as a given and the procreative process as natural (1983:107).

The similarity between conservative and radical feminist positions is their desire to locate femininity in the body. Socialist feminist arguments on the other hand assume that femininity is something "given to the body" through institutions that give specific meanings to acts such as breastfeeding. In North America in the seventies, a new meaning of breastfeeding emerged. Breastfeeding an infant in a park in Florida or a shopping mall in Toronto becomes a political act when it is made part of a legal discourse about nudity, obscenity, and legal rights. In Canada, refusing INFACT permission to display brochures at a La Leche League conference and denying them discounts for bulk mail on the grounds that they are a political action group are part of the same discourse.

Of course, to a medical professional, natural has yet a third meaning—that women can breastfeed with no difficulties and there are no barriers or obstacles to this natural activity. If it is natural, then health professionals have no responsibility for providing assistance with breastfeeding. But the role of the health professional is a complex story that will be developed in the next chapter on medicalization.

Liberal and radical feminist positions also coincide in that they both advocate the removal of discriminatory constraints on women based on their reproductive processes. Technological innovations that free women from these constraints are interpreted positively in both paradigms—but for vastly different reasons. Both the liberal and radical positions can be used in support of bottle feeding, one part of the reproductive process that can be dispensed with at present. The infant formula companies appeal to these logical positions in their claims to liberate women from the drudgery of breastfeeding. Ironically, they can hardly claim to be emancipating North American and

European women—for the trend toward increased breastfeeding is occurring in North America and Europe at a time when the feminist movement is gaining credibility and momentum, and when more women are entering the work force (Winikoff 1978:898).

Feminist philosophies generate divergent opinions on other issues of interest to women such as pornography. A conservative might hold that pornography is immoral, and moral values should regulate both public and private life. A liberal might choose to stay neutral, arguing for freedom of sexual expression and a private personal response to pornography. For both liberals and Marxists, pornography may be "off the map of male politics" (Eisenstein 1983:127). It is the radical feminists who identify pornography as sexist propaganda and relate it to rape and sexual abuse. They view pornography as a symbol of patriarchy that must be destroyed; radical feminists are more likely to set fire to pornographic bookshops than to support legal censorship (Jaggar 1983:283–286). Socialist feminists are less clear on this issue. They share with radical feminists the assumption that pornography encourages the treatment of women as sex objects. However, they recognize that pornography must be linked to broader institutions of society, including the capitalist market system supplying sexual services.

Pornography, like breastfeeding, can be interpreted from a number of different feminist positions that lead to different political actions. The same rhetoric and metaphors may be used by different groups, providing a basis for occasional joint action and statements that gloss over the underlying contradictions between very different logical models.

The emotional fervor generated by the breast-bottle controversy brought to light problems that many groups would rather keep obscure in order to hold together shaky coalitions and balance conflicting interests between institutions in western society involved in infant feeding. There are a number of reasons for this beyond the philosophical assumptions underlying different feminist positions on infant feeding. Infant feeding is an emotionally loaded personal issue, and a woman's response to it is strongly influenced by her personal experience with breastfeeding or bottle feeding. Raphael, whose arguments are outlined below, documents how her own personal failure at breastfeeding changed her forever (1976). I have tried to reflect on my personal biases regarding infant feeding in the introductory chapter.

Ironically, divisions among pro-breastfeeding and pro-bottle feeding women were strengthened by feelings of guilt and shame induced in part by increased attention on breastfeeding. Knowing that "breast is best" and then choosing to bottle feed can arouse emotions of guilt or shame in North American women. Fisher distinguishes between guilt, a judgment of wrongdoing, and shame, the judgment that we have failed to live up to some ideal (1984:189–191). A number of writers have expressed the distress they felt when they failed to live up to some ideal, perhaps unmedicated natural childbirth, or the La Leche League standards of breastfeeding on demand, or "natural mothering" (McCaffery 1984; Blackman 1981).

Gerlach (1980) has described INFACT as a social movement. Like all social movements, it depends on a shared ideology, sense of purpose, and strong commitment. It is important that such social movements do not contribute to women's feelings of guilt, shame, or inadequacy concerning their choice of infant feeding methods. Fisher warns us that:

> As a social movement gains strength, this sense of liberation from imposed ideals contributes to feelings of empowerment, especially the feeling that by freeing ourselves from the oppressor's ideals we need never again be ashamed. But this sense of freedom does not take into account the way in which a movement develops its own ideals and participants impose them on each other and themselves. (1984:193)

Organizations such as INFACT and IBFAN, as well as advocacy groups, have avoided this problem by focusing on institutions and the economic context of marketing breastmilk substitutes rather than the infant feeding decisions of individual mothers. But breastfeeding support groups and industry critics are vulnerable to criticisms from women's groups for a number of reasons. One is that many women have been disillusioned by their own breastfeeding experience; they expected it to be "natural," enjoyable, or even sensually pleasurable (Minchin 1985:243), and were angered when they found that this was not true. This problem of overromanticizing breastfeeding and underplaying the difficulties many North American women face in western medical settings is a dilemma and may have cost INFACT real feminist support.

Other attacks came from industry apologists and were published in medical, nutritional, and anthropological literature, presenting what Minchin calls "an American feminist position." She, however, finds it "hard to see them as true feminists because they are so uncritically accepting of pressures that harm both mother and child" (Minchin 1985:253). This literature, widely endorsed and circulated by infant formula manufacturers, comes primarily from the Human Lactation Center and Dana Raphael. In addition to writing in the *Lactation Review,* Raphael entered into a debate in the *Journal of Nurse-Midwifery,* arguing that industry critics who press for legislation to regulate the promotion of infant formula in developing countries are really trying to restrict women's freedom to choose. Raphael argues that the WHO/UNICEF Code proposes to legislate breastfeeding and perpetuate the notion that women in the developing countries have an obligation to breastfeed. She accused Douglas Johnson, the National Chairman of INFACT, of supporting "legislation which would control the lives of poor women" (Raphael 1981:41), an argument that makes it obvious why Bristol-Myers and Nestlé purchased and circulated so many copies of the Center's publication, *Lactation Review*. Clarkson's analysis (1983) of the Human Lactation Center's tax statements revealed that 94 percent of its income in 1979–1980 came from the infant formula industry. In 1978, Raphael characterized her 1973 statement—that "a growing trend away from breastfeeding infants and towards the use of artificial milk or animal milk is resulting in increased malnutrition and death"—as an "unscientific and inaccurate statement from an individual assuming an advocate's role based on the statements of others and her own limited impressions" (1978:1). From 1978 on, the views of Raphael and the *Lactation Review* increasingly converged with those of the infant formula industry, although the industry identifies her as an independent authority. The full range of Raphael's arguments against the activists is not an issue here. The key point is that her work is presented as feminist and pro-women based on the argument that women should have the right to feed their infants any way they choose and that the WHO/UNICEF Code infringes on this freedom of choice. By not examining the broader institutional and political contexts within which infant feeding decisions are made, industry advocates have used Raphael's work as evidence that the infant formula industry is "feminist" in its support for women's right to choose how they want to feed their infants.

During the last few decades, lactation has moved out of the consciousness of North American women. The words of a famous guru of child care—"Let no mother condemn herself to be a common or ordinary cow unless she has a real desire to nurse" (Hardyment 1983:95)—must be understood in the context of rapid changes in the power of the medical profession and the growth of the infant food industry around the turn of the century. Many women no longer know how to think or talk about breastfeeding. For them, the most articulate voices, La Leche League and INFACT, must seem to be speaking two foreign languages—disturbing languages harkening back to some vague murmurings deep in their consciousness about something that was once understood but now forgotten. The words may well be more easily ridiculed than turned in upon. When women do tune into these vague murmurings—the submerged discourse about their power to nurture—they may well find they have no words, models, or metaphors for expressing this intimate power without appearing to defend biological determinism. They are thus easily muted by the forces of medical hegemony and corporate interests, the subjects explored in the following two chapters.

CHAPTER FOUR

Medicalization and the Infant Formula Controversy

THE INFANT FORMULA CONTROVERSY reflects "the costs of inscribing civilization" on women's bodies (O'Neill 1985:11). The bodily alienation that produces great levels of anxiety in western women is intimately connected with the dominance of the medical profession and its world view. The jurisdiction of the medical profession has expanded to include infant feeding in both developed and developing countries. It is now taken for granted that anything affecting infant health belongs in the medical domain. For that reason, the health professions must be intimately involved in the infant formula controversy. Health professionals are involved with infant feeding decisions both at the level of doctor-patient interaction and at the lofty heights of international health policy. Medical knowledge, institutions, and practitioners are powerful determinants of infant feeding patterns. But as we examine the infant formula controversy, it becomes clear that the role of the medical profession in the controversy is far from consistent—some would say, far from admirable.

In this chapter, I examine the role of the health professions in the infant formula controversy and lay out some of the multiple paths of influence from health professionals to infant feeding decisions. The key concept for understanding the complexity of medical influences on infant feeding is medicalization.

Medicalization of infant feeding refers to the expropriation by health professionals of the power of mothers and other caretakers to determine the best feeding pattern of infants for maintaining maximum health. There follows from this definition no judgment as to how medicalization of infant feeding relates to infant morbidity and mortality—only an argument that what was in the past largely the concern of mothers and women is increasingly part of the medical domain.

This focused question on the medicalization of infant feeding is part of the larger problem, defined by Ivan Illich in *Medical Nemesis* (1976) as the medicalization of everyday life. By this process, the medical community creates a market for its services by redefining certain events, behavior, and problems as disease; thus anxiety, obesity, alcoholism, addiction, homosexuality, and other human experiences were redefined as medical problems. (Freidson 1970; Zola 1972; Conrad and Schneider 1980). Medicalization became possible because of the growth in prestige, dominance, and jurisdiction of the medical profession. The process was facilitated by the founding of medical associations to professionalize medicine by constituting and controlling the market for medical expertise, eliminating competition, and creating a medical monopoly (Conrad and Schneider 1986:129).

Medicalization emerged as a key ingredient in the "doctor-bashing" of social scientists during the last decade (see Ehrenreich 1978; Navarro 1976, 1981). Illich has been criticized both for the content of the concept of medicalization and for presenting the analysis as if it were a conspiracy by the medical profession. Ehrenreich responds that this is not a conspiracy but the result of the institutional structure, organization, and economics of health care systems under capitalism (1978:42). Kleinman faults Illich for "attributing the failures of the health care system solely to the machinations of the medical profession, as if it were able to operate entirely independent of its social and political context" (1980:49). Medicalization of life and medical imperialism, he argues, is overstated as a conspiracy of doctors. Is it their fault if their patients and the media view them as miracle workers? Zola (1972) writes that the medicalization of society is as much a result of medicine's potential as it is of society's wish for medicine to use that potential. This rationalization minimizes the extraordinary power of medical professionals as protectors of human life and health and, according to Navarro, ignores that fact that medical bureaucracies are servants of the dominant class (1976:118).

McKeown takes issue with Illich's arguments that "medicine does more harm than good; it breeds demands for its services and supports features of society which generate ill-health; most seriously, it diminishes the capacity of the individual to deal with his own health problems and to face suffering and death" (McKeown 1979:184–185). Illich's three premises survive these criticisms unscathed for, as one might expect from a doctor, McKeown faults him for his lack of medical knowledge—("Illich was misinformed" [1979:185])—rather than addressing Illich's underlying assumptions. To McKeown, Illich has less expert knowledge and therefore does not realize the great harm that self-medication, for example, might cause (1979:187).

In spite of all the critiques of the concept, it has moved into the social science literature as a cliché—a truth to be defended or a position to be attacked—without consensus about the process itself. In order to apply the concept to infant feeding decisions, we must first determine exactly what medicalization is as a process. Medicalization includes the following elements:

1. The power to define, label, and treat conditions shifts from self, caretaker, or family member (lay person) to a health professional (healer, nurse, physician).
2. The judgment about the appropriateness of medical definition and of treatment shifts from lay persons to health professionals. That is, both health professionals and patients assume and believe that the health professional's judgment is correct and that lay interpretation is incorrect.
3. As a result of these shifts in power and judgment, the condition under discussion is redefined as being within the medical sphere of responsibility.
4. Processes that formerly were defined as within the range of normal are redefined as medical problems requiring professional medical management, regardless of whether the profession has the capacity to deal with the problem.
5. As a result of this expanded domain, medical management requires more specialized knowledge about disease and encourages new initiatives for treatment. Treatments often include new technological and pharmaceutical innovations.
6. Places where treatment occurs—hospitals and clinics—become more dominant institutions, reinforcing the shift in power and judgment to health professionals.
7. Vocabulary and concepts of medical sciences become popular rhetoric and idioms for discussing problems.

Is there anything wrong with medicalization? Before considering the example of infant feeding, consider the probable consequences following from the elements of medicalization listed above:

1. Shifts in power contribute to increasing the medical monopoly over health as a commodity; rules are "given" to patients, and they are expected to comply.

2. Lay persons' understanding of their own health conditions and folk and popular medical theories are compared with biomedical models, and the former are usually devalued as less reliable, less accurate, and less effective according to the dominant biomedical explanatory model.
3. Biomedical models become "the only text in town," providing the language and terminology for talking about particular conditions. This specialized discourse is effective for communication between professionals but often mystifying to patients.
4. Health professionals are pressured to solve problems, develop treatments, and cure conditions that formerly may have been considered within the range of normal or treated by others, such as midwives or shamans, for example.
5. In search of new treatments, relations are strengthened between medical professionals and industry, as commercial companies assist in the development of technological solutions that benefit both industry and the medical profession.
6. Medical institutions become potentially more powerful institutions for promoting changes in health behaviors. In Foucault's terms, the hospital becomes a place of therapeutic action, a curing machine, and a place for the accumulation and development of knowledge for the training of doctors (1980:180–181).
7. Medicalization individualizes human problems and removes them from their social and economic contexts.

The process of medicalization is facilitated by claims published in reputable medical journals, enabling doctors to secure legitimacy and define their "turf." It is likely that the process of medicalization is also influenced by payment method. Human problems may well be defined as medical problems so that insurance programs will cover costs (Conrad and Schneider 1986:133). The following section suggest how the medicalization of infant feeding developed.

THE DEVELOPMENT OF MEDICALIZED INFANT FEEDING

In the west, infant feeding has a long history of association with medical professionals. Fildes (1986) documents in great historical detail the medical advice and practices regarding infant feeding from 1500 to 1800 in Britain and Europe. With the mid-fifteenth-century invention of printing, vernacular works on child rearing, pediatrics, and midwifery were produced. While it could be argued that pediatric and midwifery texts were directed to medical students and did not reflect lay practices, they do provide clues about current ideas and debates about infant feeding. Generally, infant feeding received less attention that diseases of infancy, and "few writers showed any interest in the techniques of breastfeeding, presumably because it was considered to be the province of women and midwives" (Fildes 1986:117). The separation between pediatrics and midwifery steadily increased from the 1730s on, as "books on paediatrics and infant management began to be published separately from texts on midwifery" (Fildes 1986:134). This historical development is no surprise to western women who find that lactation, part of the domain of both pediatrics and obstetrics, often becomes the responsibility of neither.

Wet-nursing was popular among wealthy English women from 1500 to 1700, when even middle-class women hired wet nurses. During the eighteenth century, the trend toward early maternal breastfeeding contributed to a decline in infant mortality and maternal morbidity and mortality from milk fever. This shift was facilitated by the growing recognition of the value of colostrum, which was used almost as a purge and required putting the infant to the mother's breast shortly after birth (Fildes 1986:83). But around the same time, medical acceptance of artificial feeding increased (Fildes 1986:79). However, the domain of supplementary feeding generally continued to be outside the realm of interest and expertise of both physicians and midwives and considered the province of women. "Quite simply, men did not know, and did not regard it as their concern" (Fildes 1986:252). It became their concern, however, in the nineteenth century, when infant foods began to be produced commercially. "In the late nineteenth century in North America, medical practitioners did not have a monopoly on infant-feeding advice. A mother might turn to a physician for recommendations on 'bringing up the baby by hand,' but she also had other sources—friends, relatives, periodicals and the manufacturers of infant foods—from which she could learn about bottle feeding" (Apple 1980:404). But by the early twentieth century, with the growth of pediatrics as a specialty, parents were directed to the physician to oversee "medically-directed infant feeding" as a part of preventative medicine (Apple 1980:408). As mothers turned to patent baby foods, they could follow the instructions themselves without medical supervision, an economically harmful practice for the physician. By 1910, several companies shifted their marketing and advertising of patent infant foods away from consumers and to the physicians; they also removed directions from the package, recommending instead that mothers see their physician. The companies stressed that in this way infant feeding would be brought under the control of the medical profession. For example, in 1924 Nestlé introduced Lactogen, "sold only on the prescription or recommendation of a physician" (Apple 1980:412). Pediatricians recognized the dangers of artificial feeding of infants, but these dangers simply increased the need for medical supervision of the task and strengthened the relation between industry and the medical profession. "Manufacturers sold but medical practitioners controlled: a mutually advantageous relationship between physicians and infant food companies had been established" (Apple 1980:417).

One mutually beneficial relationship between pediatricians and industry developed in the 1930s at the Hospital for Sick Children in Toronto. There, Drs. Tisdall and Drake were involved in the search for the perfect infant food to reduce infant morbidity from infections. They developed two special products, Sunwheat biscuits and Pablum. Rights to produce the biscuit were sold to Loblaw's, a prominent chain of grocery stores in Canada; those for Pablum were awarded to the Mead Johnson company in Chicago, with royalties going to support further research on child health at the Hospital for Sick Children (Collar 1978). Ironically, the hospital stopped serving Pablum for several years, because Mead Johnson altered the original recipe by adding sugar, salt, and vegetable oil. The relationship between physicians and the infant food industry has a long history, and it has strongly influenced professional responses to the infant formula controversy, as we shall see later in this chapter.

Medicalization in the Developing Countries

Is infant feeding less completely medicalized in third world countries? Biomedical western physicians are not the only or the first health specialists to pay special attention to infants and children. Pediatrics was a well-developed medical specialty in the Ayurvedic tradition of ancient India, judging from the earliest works of medicine to survive (1500–800 B.C.) (Fildes

1986:13). The humoral traditions throughout the world are used to adjust the heating and cooling properties of foods and medicines to balance the health of even the most vulnerable family members, infants, and children. Is infant feeding medicalized in these traditions? Not completely, according to the criteria developed earlier, for infant feeding decisions are not professionalized: mothers and caretakers adjust feeding decisions themselves according to culturally determined standards of appropriateness of foods.

Biomedical therapies and institutions in developing countries often were established under colonial or neocolonial conditions, bringing essentially foreign concepts into the health field. Their very "foreignness" resulted in greater distancing between physicians and their patients, who were likely to be operating from very different explanatory models. The greater the disjunction between indigenous medical knowledge and the imported biomedical theories, the greater the efforts of local physicians to debase traditional, indigenous, "folk" medical models in order to legitimize themselves to their foreign teachers. By "emulating their oppressors," the physicians developed local health care systems based on the model of western systems. These efforts were supported by identifiable linkages between western and nonwestern countries. Many of these linkages are still in place.

How were these medical institutions linked? In many countries, local doctors were trained in European or North American hospitals, particularly for postgraduate and specialist training. Later generations favored these foreign-trained doctors and encouraged lineages of doctors trained at the same institution. Contacts were maintained through consultancies that brought foreign doctors to Europe or North America for extra training and western consultants to foreign countries for planning and evaluation missions (see Higginbottom 1984 for a discussion of psychiatry in Southeast Asia).

In countries like Thailand, medical education received substantial support from groups such as the Rockefeller Foundation, which developed a curriculum that followed western standards; no attempt was made to integrate indigenous theories or practitioners into this program. Donaldson writes that "the differentiation of modern medical professionals from the group of traditional healers occurred as a result of the development of Siriraj Hospital and medical school under Rockefeller Foundation auspices" (1981:120). It is ironic that in the last decade, international health organizations have argued for the integration of indigenous therapies and practitioners into health care delivery systems.

Medicalized infant feeding is an important part of the health adaptation system in third world cities where hospitals and western-trained physicians are concentrated. It would be a mistake to assume that the process of medicalization is identical in all developing countries, or indeed, identical to the process in the west. Some degree of creative accommodation occurs with indigenous theories, therapies, and practitioners. With reference to the attributes of medicalization defined earlier, the process of medicalization in developing countries may differ in predictable ways. The power and authority of the physician may be greater in developing countries, although the western-style physician may be only one of several alternative experts consulted for medical problems. Although many mothers may do what they are told, there is evidence from the infant feeding study that doctors did not give mothers much advice on infant feeding before the baby was born.

Does this mean that infant feeding is not always viewed as within the medical domain? While doctors may assume that infant feeding is still the domain of mothers, mothers are increasingly impressed with physicians as a source of supplies and information about breastmilk substitutes. It is not the domain of infant feeding that has become medicalized in third world countries but the more specialized domain of artificial feeding. Because breastfeeding is still considered the domain of women and midwives, physicians and mothers interact primarily in the arena of artificial feeding and health problems of mothers and infants.

When third world health professionals are cut off from indigenous knowledge of lactation management, traditionally the domain of women and midwives, they become even more dependent on the therapies and treatments developed by industry. New marketing opportunities for infant foods and pharmaceuticals coincided with physicians' needs for new management strategies for problems related to infant feeding in both developed and developing countries. These problems include lactose-intolerant and preterm infants, the newest target populations for special infant formula. These commercial solutions further ensure that infant feeding remains part of the medical domain in industrial, developed countries, and increasingly in developing countries as well.

Talking about Infant Feeding

Almost invariably in North America and increasingly in developing countries, the medicalization of infant feeding has resulted in the domination of biomedical language, knowledge, and theories for interpreting infant feeding over other modes of discourse. Press argues that "biomedical jargon is designed to allow standardized teaching of medicine and standardized communication between medical professionals. It is not designed for physician-patient interaction" (1982:191). The physician's use of this jargon with patients establishes professional legitimacy and theoretically educates patients about biomedical definition, standards, and understanding of infant feeding. Illich, of course, has a different interpretation: "The religious preference given to scientific language over the language of the layman is one of the major bulwarks of professional privilege. The imposition of this specialized language upon political discourse about medicine easily voids it of effectiveness" (1976:255).

Terms such as "colostrum," "engorgement," and the "insufficient milk syndrome," which are derived from biomedical models, influence the way mothers think about infant feeding. For many, the terms and their translations may mystify more than clarify the process of lactation.

Where infant formula is a new product, it may well be reassuring for mothers to learn of its proteins and vitamins, or even its plasma amino acid patterns. This analysis of the constituents of milks is clearly derived from the biochemical foundations of the biomedical model and emphasizes the comparability of infant milks, making it easier for professionals and mothers to assume that human and artificial milks are equivalent.

The biomedical explanatory model may motivate the decision that mothers in western countries make to breastfeed their infants. They have easy access to medical-evidence arguments that breastmilk as a product has desirable properties and contains valuable nutrients. They can compare this with the composition of other milk products and make their "rational" choice accordingly. On the other hand, the resurgence of breastfeeding in the west may have been more motivated by a process-oriented approach to health and life styles where breastfeeding fits with natural childbirth and health foods. Both interpretations are probably present in the same community or in the mind of one mother. But the product interpretation of breastfeeding is more compatible with the transmission of biomedical information in clinics and hospitals and is reinforced by industry information and advertisements.

Most research on infant feeding is based on the biomedical model of infant feeding, a model based on current experimental and clinical evidence, reported in medical journals, and taught through medical texts and medical schools. It is this "scientifically correct" knowledge about infant feeding that is usually tested in knowledge and belief questions on health surveys. The logic behind these questions is "How many of the scientifically correct answers to my questions do you know? How much of my truth do you also recognize as truth?" This research method assumes that the scientific "truth" is known, and known by doctors, and that when respondents check the "right answer," they do so for the "right" reasons—i.e., they use the same logic as biomedical specialists for coming to their decision to check "agree." The effect of this research strategy is to expand the biomedical discourse about infant feeding, masking differences in interpretation and logic that may underlie infant feeding decisions. These research strategies further strengthen medical hegemony.

Hegemony and Medical Monopoly

In analyzing psychiatry in the third world, Higginbotham outlines how "professionalism artifically circumscribes the pool of indigenous helpers available to a people by defining certain human conditions as requiring professional solutions" (1984: 29). But at the same time that international health organizations are advocating the deprofessionalization of primary care as the most important step in raising national health levels (Newell 1975), in the industrialized countries, medical bureaucracies are engaged in protecting their boundaries from encroachment by paraprofessionals and alternative healers such as naturopaths and chiropractors.

It is tempting to blame western medical practitioners and facilities for the increasing use of breastmilk substitutes in the world—and to idealize non-western practitioners. Eisenberg and Kleinman point out that this romanticism leads to an overvaluation of the skills of traditional healers and a reverse ethnocentrism against biomedical health care professionals (1981:11). Traditional healers constantly modify their beliefs and practices and cannot, of course, be considered a homogeneous group. They do not represent a single unified "traditional" view; nor are they or their treatments universally supportive of practices resulting in optimal infant feeding. For example, traditional healers in Thailand and Indonesia may have perpetuated the idea that colostrum or "the first milk" is impure and unsuitable for newborns. They also encourage feeding early solids such as rice and bananas. The practice of withholding breastmilk when infants are sick is supported by reference to traditional humoral theories of disease in both Southeast Asia and Colombia. However, the germ theory of disease causation is increasingly being substituted to perpetuate ideas that infants and mothers should be separated after birth to prevent infections.

On the other hand, traditional Javanese midwives encourage successful breastfeeding through the provision of personal services such as massages after childbirth and preparation of herbal tonics (jamu). Even mothers delivering in Semarang hospitals use the services of traditional healers on their return home. These midwives are usually less familiar with artificial feeding and unlikely to be suitable targets for promotional activity from infant formula salespersons. In Semarang, the traditional midwives were considered of too low status for the salespersons to bother with.

It is sound anthropological practice to investigate the role of traditional healers, their theories, and pratices before generalizing about their likely affect on infant feeding practices. Do we, however, assume too much about biomedical health professionals' knowledge about infant feeding?

What if the knowledge base for "medicalized infant feeding"

were incomplete, narrower than the indigenous knowledge base, based on "incorrect" assumptions, or influenced by commercial vested interests? Then real contradictions could exist between the knowledge of infant feeding possessed by women and traditional healers and the knowledge of infant feeding informing doctors' advice. This is clearly a question to be explored rather than a statement of fact. However, surveys in Kenya on the knowledge of health workers in Kenya concluded that there was "a definite lack of knowledge among health workers particularly about the mechanisms of lactation, but to some extent also about the advantages of breastfeeding" (Veldhuis et al. 1982:29).

From Process to Problem

Medicalization carves medical problems and diseases out of what were formerly defined as deviant, morally wrong, or natural processes within the range of normal rather than pathogenic occurrence. Again, medicalization may be beneficial or detrimental to infant health. A beneficial redefinition concerns the medicalization of diarrhea. To many Thai and Javanese mothers, infant diarrhea is an inevitable, natural condition that marks normal stages in an infant's development—teething, crawling, and walking, for example. Through health education, mothers are coming to "medicalize" diarrhea, defining it not as a normal condition but as a symptom requiring medical management or home remedy. Amporn was advised by her doctor to put salt in a bottle of Sprite to cure her infant's diarrhea. The medicalization of infantile diarrhea would be beneficial if mothers continued to breastfeed and intervened with oral rehydration salts. But Grace and her neighbors in Kibera, Nairobi, treated the oral rehydration salts as a medicine to prevent diarrhea. Unfortunately, many Bangkok mothers are likely to "treat" infant diarrhea by shifting to a new brand of infant formula, assuming that the diarrhea was caused by breastmilk or by the "wrong" brand of infant formula.

Medicalization of a process such as lactation has had very different results. To begin with, doctors in North America are unlikely to study the process of normal lactation, but rather study breast abnormalities and problems. They place less emphasis on breastfeeding management than on learning the composition of artificial formula. Chetley cites a study of 742 nursing schools around the world that found that the significance of breastmilk was rarely covered in the curriculum (1986:10).

The process of normal lactation includes fluctuations in milk production to meet changing demands of growing infants; it also reflects mothers' health and emotional states. Changes in supply and demand are part of the natural process of lactation and are not medical problems as such. Medicalization encourages labeling and redefining parts of these natural states as medical problems. In the first example, identifying insufficient milk as a syndrome (Gussler and Breisemeister 1980) labels and medicalizes the low point in the process of producing milk. This labeling benefits doctors, who no longer need to monitor the background conditions influencing their lactating patients. Doctors regain control over their patients by labeling their disease and providing them with a treatment that removes the symptoms. In our study, the treatment was often infant formula. Health professionals are expected to prescribe cures, not reduce stress or give social support to patients. It is also not uncommon for health professionals to encounter a situation in which a mother who claims that she has no breastmilk is found, upon a brief examination, to have copious amounts (Greiner, Van Esterik, and Latham 1981; Van Esterik 1988). This may account for the tendency among some medical practitioners to consider insufficient milk as a psychosomatic problem. Medicalizing the insufficient milk syndrome also benefits infant formula companies who can capitalize on a mother's concern about the quality and quantity of her milk supply through advertisements to health professionals. The identification of the insufficient milk syndrome is a "legitimate" reason for promoting their products. The medical labeling of the syndrome encourages the industry to provide a solution to the problem, a cure for the syndrome. It is not in their interests to be concerned that their products often cause the syndrome in the first place.

Promotion of breastmilk substitutes can influence insufficient milk in at least three ways:

> First, "insufficient milk" can result from infant food company promotional activities that undermine a mother's confidence in the quality or quantity of her own milk, especially when these promotional efforts are channeled via trusted health professions. Second, promotional activities can help create and extend socially held beliefs about the likelihood of a woman suffering from "insufficient milk." Again, this can be especially powerful if health professionals as well as mothers are anxiously waiting for the slightest sign of "insufficient milk." Third, infant food companies can extend the availability and awareness of their products to ever wider markets. This is often combined with promotional activities to ensure that the response to "insufficient milk," when perceived, is to supplement with infant formula rather than attempt to incrase the volume of breast milk. (Greiner, Van Esterik, and Latham 1981:241)

The second example of medicalization concerns the labeling of nipple problems. Women's breasts and nipples come in a variety of sizes and shapes. In spite of *Playboy* images, there is no normal breast, and no "ideal" breast shape for breastfeeding. Normal breastfeeding requires adjusting the positions of mother and infant to fit with variations in body shape. The size and shape of breasts and nipples can even be affected by clothing styles. The corsets of leather, metal, or bone that were popular in the European Middle Ages flattened the breasts. "Any woman whose nipples had a tendency to be inverted or otherwise misshapen would be further handicapped, in regard to breastfeeding, by this clothing" (Fildes 1986:102). Cecily Williams relates the rise in artificial feeding in Singapore in the 1930s to unsuitable clothing. "They have given up binding their feet because all the world agrees that it's a mutilating and unlovely procedure. But they still bind their chests so that their breasts become atrophied and useless" (1986:67).

A breastfeeding promotion campaign in Bangkok had as one of its components a breast examination clinic to identify breast and nipple abnormalities that contraindicated breastfeeding. While there are probably useful treatments to prepare inverted nipples for breastfeeding, there is also a wealth of practical knowledge about adjusting positions of mother and infant—knowledge that is easily transmitted only when breastfeeding is prevalent and public. It is unlikely that this knowledge is effectively transmitted to health professionals. Because of this discontinuity between women's and traditional midwive's practical knowledge of lactation management and the physician's definition of medical problems, health professionals turned elsewhere for solutions to these newly defined problems of medical management, such as the "dreaded" insufficient milk syndrome and abnormal nipples.

It is convenient that the pharmaceutical industry can provide solutions for medically labeled conditions. Labeling of anxiety neurosis coincides nicely with the development of Valium and other tranquilizers. Ritalin for hyperactive children, Depo-Provera for sexual disorders, and Methadone for heroin addiction provide profitable relief from more complex social problems. Chronic pain centers reinforce the need for a variety of pain killers. Infant formula manufacturers are both the cause and the cure for the insufficient milk syndrome. The transformation of the natural fluctuations in breastmilk production into a medical problem by labeling the low production point as a disease further reinforces the need for breastmilk substitutes. Infant formula becomes a convenient solution for a newly defined medical problem, a point subtly stressed in advertising copy.

Technological Solutions

To improve medical management of infant feeding, doctors turned to technological solutions. This is by no means a recent phenomenon or limited to infant feeding. Equipment to facilitate breastfeeding dates from at least the mid-fifteenth century and includes, glass breast pumps, sucking glasses, and nipple shields of tin, lead, pewter, silver, horn, bone, ivory, wood or glass (Fildes 1986:141–147). "Absent," short, or inverted nipples were "treated" with nipple shields. An advertisement for a nineteenth-century nipple shield reads: "The Medical Professional strongly advise that ALL MOTHERS should use a Breast Shield, especially during the first week of Nursing as a protection against the pain arising from tender nipples" (Minchin 1985:144). Commenting on the advertisement, Minchin writes: "Note, too, the invocation of the blessing of the medical profession, which has been an essential selling strategy for every dangerous new innovation in infant feeding" (1985:145).

With saturation marketing of infant foods and drugs in third world cities, consumers have very high expectations about instant cures. Third world doctors, who have no mandate to relieve poverty nor any firsthand experience with programs to alleviate poverty, can offer only western products to restore health. Even knowing that the root cause of illness and malnutrition is poverty, they are not trained to offer solutions at either the individual or the community level. Physicians in cities like Bangkok and Nairobi face patients with even higher expectations about "instant" cures and "supermedicines" than patients in North America. Latham links this dilemma to the attitude that "if you have a problem, all you need is a technological fix," perpetuated by a medical profession conditioned to "an assumption of the intrinsic superiority of technologic solutions," in the context of industries "ready to make a huge profit with little concern for the problems of the consumer" (1978:429).

The more effort a society expends to produce or import infant formula, the more effort will be expended to use the product and the greater the belief that the product will bring health to infants. For many women in Bangkok, the key infant feeding problem is the need to ensure increased quantities of infant formula, certainly not to question the utility or worth of the product.

Pfifferling argues that "technology increases iatrogenic risk and the social distance between doctor and patient" (1981: 213). Although we are used to thinking of medical technology in terms of scanners, dialysis machines, and other costly and complex machinery, the statement applies equally well to infant feeding bottles and commerical infant foods in low-income households and communities.

Hospitals and Clinics

Medicalization strengthens the influence of hospitals and clinics as places where infant feeding decisions are negotiated. They can therefore have a potentially powerful influence on mothers through routines and practices favorable to either breastfeeding or bottle feeding and through direct promotion of one or the other methods of feeding.

The importance hospitals and clinics have in decisions regarding infant feeding depends on the extent to which infant feeding is medicalized. If it is not, if the hospital is merely the location where doctors work, then hospital influence will be less important. If infant feeding is medicalized, then the influence of the institution may be substantial. But again, the influence may be mobilized to support either breastfeeding or bottle feeding.

Hospitals may have an even greater influence on infant feeding decisions in developing countries than in North America. Hospitals, a product of the biomedical model of health care, developed in the west as doctors' workshops—they were places for teaching physicians and for research as well as locations for curing activities. This expensive model of hospital-based health services was effectively transplanted into developing countries (Rifkin 1985:3). Illich's descriptions of nineteenth-century hospitals reflects how hospitals are viewed in developing countries—museums of disease and places of death (1976:162). Nevertheless, hospitals are the main focus for delivery of health care services in most developing countries. Illich writes:

> All countries want hospitals, and many want them to have the most exotic modern equipment. The poorer the country, the higher the real cost of each item on their inventories. Modern hospital beds, incubators, laboratories, respirators, and operating rooms cost even more in Africa than their counterparts in Germany or France where they are manufactured: they also break down more easily in the tropics, are more difficult to service, and are more often than not out of use. (1976:56)

For women in developing countries, hospitals may seem unfamiliar, unfriendly, and frightening places. Nevertheless, according to women responding to the infant feeding survey, nearly all births in Bangkok and Bogotá, 86 percent of Nairobi births, and 55 percent of births in Semarang took place in hospitals or clinics.

Nairobi. Grace gave birth at home in Kibera, assisted by a neighbor. Elsewhere in Nairobi, private hospitals compete for deliveries of middle- and upper-class women. These mothers treat the hospital like a hotel and expect the hospital to meet all of the needs of their infants. Here, according to one nursing sister, "babies are treated as hospital property." Although 80 percent of mothers who delivered in health care facilities had their newborns in the same room with them, 38 percent of these infants were fed with infant formula or glucose solutions. Thus, in Nairobi rooming-in cannot be said to promote exclusive breastfeeding. Infants delivered in Nairobi hospitals and infants delivered by health professionals were more likely to be given infant formula (58 percent) compared with mothers like Grace delivering at home (37 percent). Overall, hospital births in Nairobi were associated with a decreased tendency to breastfeed for six or nine months' duration, regardless of background and employment factors. Even in rural areas, the association between hospital delivery and use of infant formula holds true, as Cosminski found among the Luo of South Nyanza in Western Kenya (1985:41).

Less than half of the Nairobi mothers receiving prenatal care recall being given any advice on infant feeding, and nearly one-third of these mothers were either misinformed or uninformed. Of the 757 mothers giving birth in health facilities, only 14 percent recall being given any information on infant feeding. Of these, three-fourths left the hospital with wrong information or partial information. Of all mothers delivering in health care facilities, nearly one-fourth felt that the health workers preferred either exclusive bottle feeding or a combination of breastfeeding and bottle feeding. In fact, 8 percent of mothers recalled health workers suggesting a particular brand of infant formula to them (most often the Nestlé products, Nan and Lactogen).

Bogotá. In the social security hospitals of Bogotá, mothers on social security receive four cans of infant formula per month for six months if their infants have a medically recognized nutritional need. Mothers of babies born in these hospitals are more likely to introduce an early bottle and the least likely to breastfeed. But women like Rosa, who do not receive the social security benefits associated with formal employment, must purchase the expensive products themselves or receive them as gifts. Women using health services after childbirth received recommendations for specific brands of infant formula from their physicians. These recommendations reinforced concerns over the quality of their breastmilk. Rosa followed her doctor's advice and his recommendations about the amount to feed and gave her twins S-26 when she could afford it.

A few Bogotá mothers (6 percent) received free samples of infant foods from hospitals. In spite of the high percentage of women with rooming-in (87 percent), this did not stop them from taking their physician's advice to begin using infant formula when their babies were very young. They were convinced that their breastmilk was inadequate to meet their infants' needs.

Semarang. Indonesian health centers have a long tradition of distributing free or cheap milk supplies for infants. In 1939, infant welfare centers in Batavia (Jakarta) supplied milk at reduced cost. The Dutch advisers wrote, "Artificial feeding is more often required than was formerly supposed and in many cases it is indispensable" (Hesch 1948:124). They complimented the School of Medicine at Batavia for its excellently equipped milk distribution centers where lactic acid milk was prepared and distributed to infants in the urban villages (Hesch 1948:125). Sutedjo (1974) documents six well-baby clinics in the late thirties where diluted milk in bottles was distributed to mothers unable to breastfeed.

In the fifties, the distribution of free powdered milk was an inducement to attend maternal and child health clinics, and there were fears among the staff that UNICEF milk would run out. There was also bulk milk powder selling on the black market in Javanese cities (Freedman 1955:36). The World Food Program (WFP), WHO and UNICEF continue to supply milk powder for distribution to government maternal and child health clinics throughout Indonesia as an incentive to bring mothers to the clinics. Unlike industry products which are in cans, "WFP milk products are dispensed in plastic sacks closed by an elastic band without a single word or diagram explaining proper mixing and with no measuring instrument provided. The result is predictable: improperly mixed often heavily contaminated bottle feeds, a reduction in lactation, and a new level of dependency upon the health services for infant food supplies" (Rohde 1982:172). Sutedjo raised another important point: "older infants (over one year) are seldom brought to the centre unless the distribution of skim milk takes place. . . . One wonders if the milk is consumed by children or sold by parents to purchase rice for the family" (1968:258).

One urban health center studied in Semarang received UNICEF milk powder through the city health office, but the distribution was not regular—sometimes once a month, sometimes one in three months. When the powdered milk was not available, samples of Lactona, locally made infant formula, were given to needy children instead. The distribution was directed to anemic pregnant women and to malnourished children. Those under one year received a mixture of skim milk and full cream milk, while children between the ages of one and five received skim milk only.

The mothers in central Semarang knew that it was possible to get free infant food when it was distributed by certain trading companies through sales promotion. It is difficult to estimate how five decades of free milk powder distribution in local health centers has influenced mothers' understanding of breastmilk substitutes. Certainly it has increased the availability and knowledge of such products. Both skim milk powder and full cream powder are referred to as *air susu buatan,* substitutes for mother's milk.

When infants were brought to health centers with diarrhea, clinic policy was to advise women to stop breastfeeding until the oral rehydration treatment had been completed. This may reinforce the idea that breastmilk causes diarrhea. Both physicians and *bidan* (trained midwives) influenced mothers to introduce bottle feeding for weaning purposes and as a response to problems of insufficient milk and breast morbidity. In the infant feeding survey, mothers who gave birth in a hospital and were attended by a physican or bidan were less likely to be breastfeeding at twelve months and more likely to introduce early bottles.

Although infant formula is not uniformly distributed at health facilities in Semarang, two cases illustrate how the health center may influence infant feeding patterns:

> Nyonya San, a middle-class Chinese mother from Kranggan Dalam, gave birth by Caesarean section at a private maternity clinic where S-26 was given to her son. She was under intensive care and could not breastfeed her son for five days. When she left for home, the hospital gave her S-26. Later she changed to Lactogen and then to Morinaga but returned to S-26 since it seemed to agree best with her baby. At three months, the baby stopped breastfeeding entirely because he developed diarrhea.
>
> Nyonya's Is's second child was born at home with the help of a traditional midwife. Her baby breastfeeds and is healthy. His health was protected by a *suwuk* ceremony at seven months. But if the baby has a fever, she takes him to her uncle for an injection. She took her baby to the health clinic at two months and was given free milk powder because the bidan said the child was sick and underweight.

These two women received milk products from health professionals: the wealthy from a private hospital to supplement her breastmilk and encourage her to choose this brand when she stopped breastfeeding; the poor from a health clinic, because the child was underweight.

Bangkok. Women in Bangkok are strongly committed to hospital births. The trend toward western-style obstetric care began in the mid-1800s when Dr. Bradley, an American medical missionary, tried to substitute western obstetrical methods for what he considered to be barbaric, life-threatening practices of the traditional Thai midwives. The control of the Thai medical curriculum by the Rockefeller Foundation further encouraged hospital-centered childbirth in urban centers. Even in rural areas, women showed a preference for western-style clinic births over traditional Thai methods (Muecke 1976).

Over 70 percent of Bangkok mothers in the study had prenatal care in public hospitals. Follwing childbirth, about half the mothers had their infants in the room with them. This early contact did not discourage early bottle use among Bangkok mothers. Since infants were bottle fed by nurses with infant formula in the hospital, it is not surprising that mothers assumed bottle feeding had medical support. In fact, 38 percent of the mothers were given a brand endorsement by a health professional.

Health professionals directly promote commercial infant feeding products when they recommend specific brands, give samples personally, or offer discounts or incentives to patients to purchase certain brands from them or from their institutions. In Bangkok, the relation between detail persons from infant formula companies and health professionals was both direct and observable. Similar strategies may have been employed in the other cities, but the ethnographers were unable to document these relations. In Bangkok, relations between detail persons and health professionals were particularly congenial because the salespersons were former nurses who used existing social networks to reach their former colleagues. Salespersons were observed in the hospital lunch room and the nurses' dormitory. The hospital is the locus of industry-medical interaction. A Bangkok retailer described her work as follows:

> Every company's detailers are all here. The detailers know the nurses working in these hospitals. Milk detailers are assigned to specific zones or groups of hospitals . . . we are here to meet doctors and nurses. . . . We cannot talk to mothers because the Ministry of Public Health prohibits us. . . . Now that the Ministry is campaigning for breastfeeding, they forbid us to make direct contact with mothers . . . so we find the way out by approaching through medical personnel. . . . Ordinarily, patients and mothers believe the words of the medical doctors—once they know the brands of formula the hospitals use they tend to follow, which is helpful to us. . . . We sell at a very special price to hospital staff like nurses and doctors. The price for these persons has to be lower than anywhere else. . . . It's a kind of persuasion, or public relations. These people are a good help to us. . . . Nurses often buy directly from detailers because they can get it cheap. They order formula for relatives and friends. All detailers are nurses with B.A. degrees. We used to work as nurses in these hospitals before. There is no rule in the hospital against the detailers. It is our right to contact doctors or nurses. (Svetsreni n.d.:71)

In Bangkok, mothers may chose health care facilities where they have a personal contact of some kind. Even a distant contact—"the sister of my friend is a nurse there"—is enough reason to choose that facility. Nurses have more direct contact with mothers, and it is easier for mothers to approach them with questions. On the other hand, nurses are also in contact with detail persons from infant formula companies and make the infant formula purchases for their wards. They are in charge of the milk supply rooms and determine how much infant formula can be sold to patients. According to a company representative who was visiting the same hospital where she had been a staff nurse, nurses make a commission of between 5 percent and 6 percent on each can of infant formula.

Free samples of infant formula were reported received from hospitals, clinics, or physicians by 12 percent of the mothers surveyed in Bangkok, 6 percent in Bogotá and Semarang, and 5 percent in Nairobi. These figures probably underestimate the number of samples distributed in other forms—nurses giving "gifts" to friends in hospitals, infant formula sold at reduced cost in hospital stores, and damaged cans ("booby tins") sold on hospital grounds at reduced prices once a week, as occurred in Bangkok.

Following the WHO/UNICEF Code of Marketing for Breast-milk Substitutes, infant food companies no longer market through "milk nurses." Instead, they hire competent health professionals who are experienced in maternal and child health to promote their products legally and directly through the health care system. In cities like Bangkok, this increases the impact of industry influences on infant feeding decisions.

Medical Professionals and the Infant Formula Controversy

With the exception of a few doctors who chose an advocate's role in the controversy (D. Jelliffe and M. Latham in the United States, Elizabeth Hillman in Canada), most doctors who spoke out on the infant formula controversy stressed the lack of adequate research and scientific evidence brought to bear on the controversy. This objective stance not only increased their scientific credibility among their colleagues but also endeared them to industry: Chetley cites pediatrician Dr. Charles May, former editor of *Pediatrics:* "no substantial, sound, scientific data were ever set forth by the critics of industry or officials of the WHO to support the claim that marketing practices for infant formulas have actually been a significant factor in decline in prevalence of breastfeeding in the Third World or anywhere else." Chetley also quotes Dr. Dugdale, head of the Human Nutrition Research Group of the Department of Child Health at the University of Queensland, as saying that "scientists should view with misgivings some aspects of the WHO Code for the marketing of breast-milk substitutes. . . . Much of the evidence for and against breast and bottle feeding is of doubtful scientific validity" (Chetley 1986:142). Dugdale argues that the assumptions underlying the WHO Code—that breastfeeding is better than other forms of feeding and that mothers in developing countries can be deluded by advertising and commercial promotion—are faulty. It is hard to believe that a physician would find fault with the assertion that breastfeeding is better than other kinds of feeding. The second assumption is not essential to the WHO Code. The code assumes that continuing commercial promotion for infant formula is not in the best interests of infant health. Dugdale, along with other critics of advocacy arguments and tactics, tries to suggest that critics of industry think that mothers are stupid, a theme repeated by the "feminist" anthropologist's argument in the last chapter. The title of the article by Dugdale that Chetley cites illustrates the medical perspective: "Breast-milk Policy Should be More Scientific" (Chetley 1986:152). Of course, the biomedical model determines the criteria for adequate research and scientific truth.

The views of medical experts are understood as being supported by balanced, objective, and dispassionate reviews of scientific evidence; the views of advocates are assumed to be unscientific and emotional. Medical professionals, however, make excuses. We hear from: "scientists who claim that all the possible avenues of research have not been explored, therefore it is too early to make a decision about what to do; people who hide behind the thought that the issue is so complex, and only part of a much larger world malaise, that it is pointless even to try to resolve it" (Chetley 1986:150). As a less than objective review states, "the specialists themselves have tended to slip away from the tangled area of scientifically determined facts to the less troublesome area of opinion" (Jayasuriya, Griffiths, and Rigoni 1984:27).

The Health Management Institute in Geneva, headed by R. Rigoni, a former vice-president of a large multinational pharmaceutical company, published an interesting critique of the breast-bottle controversy, *Judgement Reserved*. According to the authors, neither side met adequate "standards of evidence and analysis," and they identify the most important deficiencies as:

1. Misuse of statistics—careless, misleading, blatantly partisan, etc.
2. Loose epidemiological reasoning
3. Poor discrimination between formula and traditional supplements
4. Inadequate research data (sporadic, few standardized approaches)
5. Inadequate attention to maternal malnutrition syndrome
6. Insufficient milk syndrome underestimated and unresolved
7. Competing national interests underestimated
8. Sociocultural contexts ignored
9. The negative attitude and response of the health professions underestimated
10. Unfounded relationships alleged between educational level and breastfeeding
11. Overestimation of the effects of breastfeeding as a contraceptive
12. Neonatal care practices not the result of infant formula promotion

13. Inadequate use of industry's potential
14. Economic dimensions inadequately assessed
15. Control of breastmilk substitutes—inadequate evaluation (Jayasuriya, Griffiths, and Rigoni 1984:29–39).

This mixed bag of criticism and commentary stresses the advocates overgeneralization from study results, the blatant partisanship of any "scientist" supporting the advocacy position, and calls for more research on the problem, without addressing the key issues in the controversy. The authors conclude that breastmilk substitutes and supplements are indispensable to compensate for nutritional deficiencies in developing countries (Jayasuriya, Griffiths, and Rigoni 1984:41).

The opposition between the detached scientific objectivity of the medical profession and the emotional rhetoric of the advocacy campaign is most clearly argued in a Heritage Foundation publication by Carol Adelman (1983). She argues that once the emotional and political rhetoric of the controversy is stripped away, the scientific case against the infant formula companies can be reduced to five questions (1983:111). In her objective, scientific review of the evidence, which reveals uncertainties regarding the data base, she raises, and answers, the following questions:

1. Has breastfeeding declined dramatically in developing countries? (no)
2. Are bottle fed infants from the poorest families? (no)
3. Do bottle fed babies have higher disease and death rates? (no good supporting evidence)
4. Do promotional practices contribute significantly to a mother's decision to breastfeed? (evidence is not conclusive)
5. Is mother's milk the perfect food?

The question whether mother's milk is the perfect food demonstrates most clearly the selective search for evidence to support pediatricians' reluctance to offend the infant formula companies. She reviews a range of problems with breastmilk and breastfeeding, beginning with a quote from Fomon, the foremost American authority on infant nutrition, that "human milk is neither a perfect nor a complete food" (Adelman 1983:117).

Adelman concludes that the disadvantaged babies in developing countries are the victims of shoddy research and defensive public relations, and states that she hopes that in the future health and nutrition workers "will improve upon the careless and misleading use of statistics, false logic, and blatant partisanship that has characterized the infant formula debate" (1983:126). It fell to a limited number of health professionals and a large number of advocates to answer medical caution with advocacy action.

Answering physicians' questions about infant feeding research is not easy, for to be most effective, the answers must be framed within the biomedical paradigm. This gives only a partial response to the broad social, political, and ethical concerns underlying the infant formula controversy. Consider how doctors answer other doctors: Dr. Steven Joseph argues that even if random clinical trials could be carried out in developing countries, the question remains as to whether they would be ethical, given what we know about the advantages of breastfeeding (1981:384). Finally, as Joseph asks, on whom should the burden of proof lie? Minchin answers that "the onus of proof must always be upon those who want to promote or legitimise artificial substitutes for a natural product or process" (1985:3).

It is pointless to refute the evidence raised by Jayasuriya et al. and Adelman when the real argument is with the paradigm defining what questions can be asked. To attempt to do so would be to legitimize the framework of analysis they bring to the infant formula controversy. They are perfectly correct in stating the industry critics are emotional. Advocacy discourse is not meant to be unemotional or dispassionate. It is intended to draw attention to alternate ways of viewing an issue, to force recognition of the fact that something is wrong, out of balance, unjust, twisted. Objective scientific proof does not always exist on the determinants of breastfeeding, but there is certainly adequate proof to defend the superiority of breastfeeding over artificial feeding. Both sides of the controversy assembled their evidence selectively. The key questions concern who defines the questions to be asked, and who loses and benefits from the answers given.

The vested interests of the food and pharmaceutical companies and the medical profession emerge out of the medicalization of infant feeding. The relationship between physicians and the infant food industry was often evident in the heated debates during the infant formula controversy. The Protein-Calorie Advisory Group's (PAG) statement No. 23 on infant and child feeding revised in 1973 "read like a catalogue on how to improve infant formula sales . . . it was the first attempt by the industry to get an official stamp of approval for both the products and the marketing practices" (Chetley 1986:41). Pediatricians and infant formula manufacturers have had a close and productive relationship for decades. For example, in 1981, the American Academy of Pediatrics accepted a two-year contract with Abbott/Ross Laboratories, valued at $500,000 per year, for partial support of the publication *Pediatrics in Review* (Chetley 1986:114). Through financial support such as the $1.5 million for pharmaceutical advertising in the *Canadian Medical Association Journal* in 1980, the drug industry successfully convinced Canadian doctors that the interests of the industry are also those of the medical profession (Lexchin 1984:110–111).

Gifts and perks for doctors from industry probably would

have even more prestige in developing countries where so few can afford medical education. Occasional consultancies, conference invitations, and outright gifts of medical supplies take on even greater importance in areas where personal incomes and medical budgets are limited (albeit significantly greater than incomes of other professionals).

Medical associations in developing countries benefit directly from infant formula manufacturers. In 1977, for example, the Dominican Republic Medical Association received $80,000 in sales commissions on pharmaceutical products, one-half of one percent of sales. In 1981 Nestlé provided nearly $250,000 toward speakers and food at medical seminars and conventions, including the Philippine Paediatric Society (Chetley 1986:13). This link between health professionals and industry is the key to understanding the rapid medicalization of infant feeding. Minchin argues that the infant formula manufacturers' "colossal commercial interests will make them interpret reality in ways favorable to their own cause. They will be the last to accept that there are any substantial health risks inherent in a product they have been selling—they, and the researchers they have been employing" (1985:4).

Of greater concern is the question of how much infant feeding research is funded directly or indirectly by food and drug companies. In related areas where public health concerns clash with potential industrial profits, a similar pattern emerges. For example, the association of cigarette smoking with lung cancer appears valid, but some segments of the population demand absolute direct proof before accepting preventive legislation. Benarde writes:

> The only way to obtain this type of evidence would be to gather together several thousand children about age ten, divide them into two comparable groups of equal size, lock them in a stockade and observe them for several

> years, then start one group smoking while preventing the others from doing so. Since the effects of smoking are generally seen in the fifth or sixth decade of life, these two groups would be required to be under lock and key for at least forty years, under the scrutiny of scientists recording their every activity. Then, and only then, would absolute direct evidence of a cause-effect relationship be forthcoming. As this experiment is not possible, one can only wonder about the motives of those who clamor for "real" proof. (1973:20)

A cynic might also ask who funds research demonstrating the positive features of smoking. Similarly, industry benefits from the medicalization of alcoholism. According to Conrad and Schneider, "the alcoholic beverage industry, for example, vigorously supports the disease concept of alcoholism, which focuses attention on the individual drinker and away from the industry's advertising and marketing techniques" (1980:276).

The mutually beneficial arrangement between researchers and industry is reflected in the observation of a pediatrician, which appeared in an article titled the "The Role of Food Industry in Promoting Human Nutrition": he stated that "the preterm infant is perhaps the most fascinating of all the testbeds for artificial feeding" (Arneil 1983:106).

Research on the determinants of infant feeding is decidedly empiricist and informed by the biomedical model of evidence and "truth." Consequently, conscientious researchers must be cautious in concluding how promotion of infant formula, etc. affects mothers' decisions about infant feeding. Researchers fear criticisms about inappropriate research designs, false causality, and uncontrolled variables. In an effort to present the best possible case, many empiricist researchers have been too busy gathering, cleaning, and processing data to ask questions about its meaning and context within the power relations of biomedical systems. These questions are often raised from other contexts and fit most comfortably in the context of justice and consumer rights.

"Tinkering with the System"

Breastfeeding promotion is one entry point for efforts to improve infant feeding practices in North American and international communities. Promotional efforts to increase the initiation, duration, and frequency of breastfeeding include altering hospital routines, such as allowing early contact between mothers and newborns, allowing rooming-in and breastfeeding on demand, and discouraging prelacteal feeds and infant formula samples; training health professionals in lactation management; creating and supporting breastfeeding support groups; and initiating mass media campaigns. The majority of breastfeeding promotional activities are hospital centered. Campaigns are often funded from outside sources and developed by western health professionals who are well-paid consultants of Rockefeller, Ford, WHO, or bilateral aid agencies. Rarely is comparable funding given to women's breastfeeding support groups or to consumer groups who challenge the role of multinational pharmaceutical companies in hospitals and in the community. The Swedish International Development Authority (SIDA) does provide support for these groups. If groups examining structural impediments to breastfeeding, such as women's working conditions, marketing practices, and poverty environments, are not given financial and moral support, then hospital-based campaigns to promote breastfeeding are a prime example of "tinkering with the system."

In the four cities where the infant feeding study was carried out, promotion of breastfeeding was identified as part of national and institutional policy. A large government hospital in Nairobi claimed to be promoting breastfeeding and discouraging the use of infant formula. One nurse described how much work it had taken to reduce the presence of infant formula in the hospital, although younger nurses did not realize the extent of the problem in the past. In the ward for mothers delivered by Caesarean section, feeding bottles sat on the lockers in three out of four rooms, in spite of the fact that mothers had already begun breastfeeding. One mother was obviously having difficulty getting her newborn to latch on to her very short nipples, which had not been prepared for breastfeeding. The one nursing sister with breastfeeding experience showed the mother how to pull her nipples out to make them easier for her baby to grasp. The mother seemed pleased to have help, although she had not asked the sisters for assistance.

Outside a Nairobi clinic for malnourished infants where breastfeeding was promoted, a mother sat holding a small infant in a shawl. She had placed a towel over the baby and looked as though she were breastfeeding the infant; but then, when the baby stopped taking the bottle, a large rubber nipple suddenly protruded from the shawl. The mother evidently did not want the sisters to see that she was bottle feeding. Later, one nurse observed that many mothers brought a bottle of infant formula with them to the clinic, even if they were also breastfeeding. Where breastfeeding is promoted, bottle feeding is a clear disappointment and failure to the clinic personnel. The nursing sisters noted that the promotion of infant formula within the hospital was less blatant in the eighties, but felt that breastfeeding promotion campaigns were not very effective in discouraging early bottle feeding.

In a well-established private hospital in Nairobi, most of the patients were wealthy Asians. Recently, changes had been instituted to promote breastfeeding and discourage infant formula use. The Nestlé posters on child development and prenatal care hung in the hospital, but the company name and product pictures were covered over. A local breastfeeding mothers' group teaches breastfeeding management weekly and passes out information to new mothers. Yet the pediatric department's guidebook advised mothers to substitute one bottle of milk per day for breastmilk so that the baby would not come to dislike the taste of other milks. In another private hospital where breastfeeding was promoted, the local breastfeeding support group was not welcome because their advice often conflicted with the advice of the nursing staff. Outside the nursery, where mothers were reported to be encouraged to breastfeed, stood a cart of feeding bottles ready for the next delivery. Another private hospital promotes breastfeeding by having the nursing staff do all the bottle feeding so that mothers will be encouraged to breastfeed. The nurses enjoy bottle feeding newborns very much.

Breastfeeding promotion campaigns are established strategies in both urban and rural Thailand. The fifth five-year development plan for Thailand (1982–1986) included as one of its objectives maintaining full breastfeeding among 90 percent of rural mothers with infants from zero to six months. Many promotion campaigns were focused in northeastern Thailand where breastfeeding initiation rates are highest and the duration longest. A recent project targeted mainly at health professionals aimed to improve infant feeding practices at nine Bangkok hospitals through changes in hospital routines and training courses in lactation management. Initially, teams attended four-week training courses in California. On their return, these teams, which were composed of a pediatrician and pediatric nurse and an obstetrician and obstetrical nurse, set up in-country training in lactation management for their staffs. Although the intention to increase breastfeeding and decrease bottle feeding with infant formula in Bangkok hospitals was admirable, placing the emphasis on hospitals and health professionals strengthened the medicalization of infant feeding. At one large government hospital in Bangkok, breastfeeding promotion activities included a breast examination clinic to identify breast problems and abnormalities, group lectures emphasizing breastfeeding, and short "tests" of mothers' knowledge of breastfeeding. If they passed this "test," the women received a stamp on their patient chart indicating they had passed the breastfeeding course. Although the records indicate 100 percent breastfeeding rates at discharge, about half discontinue breastfeeding after one week.

Most breastfeeding promotion campaigns are conducted through hospitals and Ministries of Health, but there is some evidence that hospitals may not be the most effective places for promoting breastfeeding. In their study of community influences on breastfeeding in London hospitals, Hart et al. conclude that efforts to promote breastfeeding may prove expensive and that inevitably the hospitals cannot meet the essential requirements for successful lactation, which include:

1. A genuine commitment on the part of the mother to breastfeed. Mothers are most likely to be convinced about the merits of breastfeeding by meeting during their pregnancy mothers who have already delivered and are already lactating.
2. A relaxed environment to carry this out. A relaxed environment is best provided by the mother's own home.
3. Consistent and continuing advice during the period of time lactation is established. (Hart et al. 1980:186–187)

Hospitals may be encouraged to promote breastfeeding for the financial savings: one Bangkok hospital reported savings of 700 bottles of infant formula per day. This financial incentive is only effective if the hospital is not already receiving free supplies of infant formula.

Greiner (1982) distinguishes between policies that protect, support, and promote breastfeeding and argues that in developing countries the lowest priority should be promotion. Promotion efforts affect fewer women and are potentially least effective and least cost-effective in terms of time, money, and expertise. Promotional efforts presuppose that measures to support and protect breastfeeding are already in place. Certainly, in developing countries, efforts to protect breastfeeding by ensuring that breastmilk substitutes are not actively promoted through the health system lag far behind efforts to develop breastfeeding promotion campaigns in hospitals.

Breastfeeding promotion campaigns are ethically complex in that they infer that medical practitioners and institutions have the right to try and influence a mother's private decision about how to feed her infant. In the biomedical model, physicians have a responsibility for health education and public health, while the community should be the passive recipient of services and advice from health professionals (see Rifkin 1985). This approach to educating mothers about how to feed their infants may easily slip into moralizing and blaming mothers for their infant feeding decisions. For health professionals, breastfeeding is managed as a problem of individual patient compliance, particularly if mothers fail to breastfeed in the manner preferred by their physicians.

Navarro uses a comparable example of programs requiring individuals to change their food consumption from unhealthy to healthy foods. This avoids the question of why individuals consume the diets they do and ignores the power of corporate interests in determining food production and consumption patterns. Navarro argues that "the greatest potential for improving the health of our citizens is not primarily through changes in the behaviors of individuals, but primarily through changes in the patterns of control, structures, and behaviors of our economic and political system" (1976:128). Here we can see parallels with breastfeeding promotion campaigns that stress changes in individual attitudes and behavior of women rather than structural changes in institutions.

There are parallels between the history of the promotion of contraceptives and the promotion of breastfeeding. Both could be seen as campaigns to increase the individual freedom and choice of women; both are intimately connected with wider social and economic issues concerning production and reproduction; and both campaigns were accused by their opponents of being communist plots. The Birth Control League's campaign was "supported by Moscow gold," according to the *Boston Post,* July 25, 1916 (Gordon 1978:161). The Infant Formula Action Coalition and other advocacy groups were accused of being "Marxists marching under the banner of Christ" (Nickel 1980). Both are potentially radical feminist issues that call for structural transformations in the position and condition of women. Yet both the promotion of birth control and the promotion of breastfeeding can easily become depoliticalized and deradicalized when medical professionals take over responsibility for managing breastfeeding and birth control. Gordon argues that "birth control has failed to cross class lines because it has not been feminist enough. A feminist birth control movement would struggle to expand women's options, to extend their right to choose, not to impose a certain economic or political theory upon them" (1978:145). The involvement of the medical profession in the birth control issue turned the direction and priorities of the campaign away from feminist issues. In the early 1920s, most doctors were opposed to contraception (Gordon 1978:152). But the medical profession lent support to the birth control movement, provided they could have "exclusive control and restrictive distribution" of both contraception and contraceptive information (Gordon 1978:175).

Parallels with promotion of breastfeeding campaigns are disturbing. When male physicians define contraception or breastfeeding as a woman's duty and have a monopoly on information and management, the needs of individual women may easily be ignored. Health professionals are not always particularly sensitive or nonjudgmental with regard to contraception or breastfeeding. There is, however, one significant difference between these two campaigns. Commercial pressures are supportive of birth control, and the contraceptive business is very lucrative—over three billion dollars in 1979. But "there are no vested interests to defend breastfeeding" (Minchin 1985:193), and, as we have seen, commercial pressures on health professionals support increasing use of infant formula. As a result, campaigns to promote breastfeeding and medical endorsement for breastfeeding support groups such as La Leche League coexist with hospital routines detrimental to breastfeeding and commercial promotion of infant formula in both developed and developing countries, a situation that underscores the contradictions emerging from the medicalization of infant feeding.

Currently, medical anthropologists are seeking ways to integrate empiricist, clinical, interpretive, meaning-centred, advocacy and neo-Marxist approaches into a new critical medical anthropology. Critical medical anthropology includes broad macrostructural questions, the role of power in social life, and the way in which biomedicine is culturally constructed (Lock 1986:110). From this perspective, broader questions such as the medicalization of infant feeding can be further researched.

CHAPTER FIVE

Commoditization of Infant Food

A COMMON THEME IN THE ADVOCACY literature on the infant formula controversy is that bottle feeding and use of breastmilk substitutes have acquired meaning beyond functional value and have become status symbols in the process of westernization and modernization in third world countries. Although the argument makes good sense, it is extremely difficult to prove, partly because there is so little research on status symbols and their creation.

In 1973, Berg argued that "urbanization and modernization and new social values" are significant influences in the decline of breastfeeding. "Breastfeeding is often viewed as an old-fashioned or backward custom and, by some, as a vulgar peasant practice. . . . In most developing countries, the greater the sophistication, the worse the lactation: the bottle has become a status symbol" (1973:99). Latham also points to western influence, as "a belief develops that it is superior, chic, and sophisticated to bottle feed. Breast feeding may come to be regarded as a 'primitive' practice and the bottle become a status symbol"

(1975:iii). This symbolic interpretation as one factor in the spread of bottle feeding was further explained by the Jelliffes: "The machine-manufactured increasingly dominated as symbols of enlightenment, progress and modernness, as opposed to seemingly archaic, out-of-date traditional methods and biological practices of which breastfeeding was one" (1978:185). Bottle feeding, then, becomes an attainable symbol (Jelliffe and Jelliffe 1978:223).

CREATING STATUS SYMBOLS

What do social scientists have to say about the process of creating status symbols? Veblen's early work (1912) emphasized the nonutilitarian character of goods as status symbols. McCracken (1986) has criticized Veblen for focusing too narrowly on objects as markers of status and concentrating only on the role of goods to communicate something about status and wealth.

Baudrillard recognizes the importance of Veblen's work on the production of social classification. Although Veblen "posited the logic of differentiation more in terms of individuals than of classes, of prestige interaction rather than of exchange structure, he nevertheless offers in a way far superior to those who have followed him and who have pretended to surpass him the discovery of a principle of total social analysis, the basis of a radical logic, in the mechanisms of differentiation" (1981:76).

The marking function of consumer goods allows observers to predict something about the person possessing a particular object. Someone you know nothing about becomes slightly more knowable through his association with object X, because this association leads to certain assumptions about that person. Observers then respond to that person in terms of those assumptions. Thus, the marking function of objects is key to the creation of stereotypes.

Objects perceived as status symbols constantly change, making it difficult to count on their marking functions across subgroups and through time. It is the process of creating and generating status symbols that must be better understood. Drawing on the marking function of goods, access to an object must be restricted in some way for it to become a status symbol. Access may be restricted on the basis of the following:

1. Cost: expensive products may be self-restricting on the basis of price. Infant formula, instant coffee, etc. may first be available only at stores where the wealthy shop. Their high price puts them out of reach of low- and middle-income shoppers.
2. Rarity: only a limited number of objects available. Their restricted distribution increases their exchange and their sign value (e.g., Olympic medals and pins, marathon T-shirts, prizes from baby contests, bowling trophies, signed books, works of art, antiques, ethnic heirlooms).
3. Distance from consumer: goods imported from great distances, souvenirs from distant places, and mementos of pilgrimages from sacred places.
4. Objects associated with people of high status or presumed high status (e.g., objects once belonging to famous athletes or Hollywood stars).

In developing countries, objects associated with prestigious figures may define a category of status symbols for a class or a population. Colonial officials, medical doctors, or religious leaders may all affect the evaluations of the worth of particular objects. But neither market researchers nor social scientists are clear as to whether people emulate people of higher status or are more influenced by their peers. Barnett suggests that while the middle class is influenced by the elite, members of the lower class are more influenced by their friends (1953:315). King argues that a group will adopt behavior of the group immediately above it, not of the highest group (1964:111). Consumer researchers are well aware that their customers buy things for what they mean. The purchase of Swiss watches, when cheapter quartz imitations keep better time, is a case in point. In developing countries, the purchase and use of infant feeding bottles, Swiss watches, Pierre Cardin purses, and Coke all reflect consumers' attempts to make their environment communicate their identity as modern consumers more effectively.

The adoption of western goods in developing countries is embedded in a complex political economy. Some western objects develop almost mana-like associations—as if by contact with "ghetto-blasters," Coca-Cola, and posters of rock stars, "they" could become instantly developed like "us." The idea of power by contact is also part of the process of generating status symbols in North America: status-seekers want to touch or own something once associated with a famous event or person—moon rocks or clothing owned by a Hollywood star.

In a discussion of how the meanings of objects are produced, Gottdiener lists five ways of analyzing objects (1985:991). An object can be approached (1) physically: the material object; (2) mechanically: its instrumental or use value; (3) economically: its exchange value; (4) socially: its status or sign value; (5) semantically: its broader context with related objects. He refers to the process whereby an object develops a socially sustained sign value as transfunctionalization. In the first stage of this process, producers produce objects for their exchange value and purchasers purchase objects for their use value. In the second stage, objects are transformed and personalized by their owners to create new meanings, new sign values. Producers themselves create meanings based on the users' sign values in the third stage of meaning production. Here the role of advertising and promotion is particularly important (Gottdiener 1985).

Bourdieu, using ethnographic evidence from France, shows how struggles over the appropriation of economic or cultural goods are also struggles to appropriate distinctive signs or emblems of class. He goes much farther than other authors in identifying the source of differences in taste that differentiate groups; these dispositions toward particular food, music, art or films, for example, are acquired on the basis of social origin measured by father's occupation and education (1984:387). From this perspective, then, the meaning of objects—particularly objects that define an individual's place in the status hierarchy—is not created by the producers of the object, nor by the advertisers who popularize objects; rather, it preexists in the symbolic codes of that particular society. This is why it is harder to use objects to make boundary-crossing claims in developed countries. False claims are quickly identified as being in bad taste. In this way, the code of signification of values precedes both the functionality of goods, their use value, and individual needs. The key concepts of taste and life syle used by Bourdieu and by market researchers are rooted in the historical and cultural sign values in each community or subgroup purchasing the objects. This is why the same products may have different meanings in developed and developing countries. The sign values are derived from different cultural sources; even if the use value or exchange values is assumed to be comparable in developed and developing countries, the link between object and purchaser, the sign (or signal) value, and the context of use are most certainly very different.

The process of taste transfer for objects or foods as status symbols in developing countries might look something like this:

1. Object or food brought with colonial or expatriate household (use value)
2. Object or food imported for colonial or expatriate use
3. Object or food adopted by local elite (new sign value)
4. Demand for object or food by local middle class as status symbol
5. Larger supply becomes available (reduces currency of status symbol for local elite)
6. Local versions produced
7. Demand for object or food by low-income consumers for sign value only
8. Object or food used by middle-income consumers for use value only
9. Particular imported brand carries sign value for higher-income consumers
10. Counterfeiting or imitation of name brands occurs
11. Elite appropriate new symbols to disassociate themselves from objects or foods whose authenticity cannot be guaranteed

This cycle is further complicated by the fact that many goods that are becoming indices of status in the west are being produced in developing countries for export and only appear in local markets occasionally (when they "fall off the truck"). When they do appear, they are clearly identified as superior objects and sold as export goods at higher prices. In Bangkok shopping malls, local T-shirts compete with T-shirts for export selling for double the price. With the production of prestige items such as clothing, purses, and jewelry in developing countries, a new problem of authenticity has developed. Product markers of authenticity—a leather label, an emblematic alligator—are detached from the products they belong to and are sold in job lots to retailers and customers who reattach them to other products. Customers who purchase goods primarily for their sign value no longer can be assured of the authenticity of their purchases.

Some western goods such as plastic pails have become popular in developing countries merely because they are cheaper, more efficient, or more convenient than the local goods they replaced. They function as status symbols only when they are in restricted supply, when their meaning is derived from western countries, or when they become equated with modernization and development.

Although the process of generating status symbols is poorly understood, it is certainly clear that bottle feeding was a status symbol in the recent past and remains so in many rural areas of the developing world. To understand this process, however, it is useful to distinguish between mode of feeding and the food product. Recall that the increase in bottle feeding reflects two kinds of substitutions, one of product (breastmilk for an appropriate or inappropriate breastmilk substitute) and one of process (breastfeeding for bottle feeding). To understand the creation of status symbols, we will first examine the development of prestige foods and then consider the transfer of the bottle feeding "technology."

Delocalization and Prestige Emulation of Food

Patterns of food selection are constantly changing for both adults and infants. Explanations for some of these changes can be found in the process of commoditization. Commoditization of infant foods is the process through which infant foods (breastmilk, breastmilk substitutes, and supplementary foods) shift from being a human right with a use value embedded in complex personal relations established through shared production and consumption to being an object of exchange—a commodity based on price. Through the infant formula controversy, we have identified some of the forces behind these changes. However, Mary Douglas reminds us of the complexity underlying these shifts: "What is the direction and power that selects among the modern luxuries and processes that shift in status so that from being first unknown, then known but dispensable, some goods become indispensable" (1979:98)? Some of these selection forces are economic and reflect availability of foods, for example. But since food consumption is culturally constructed, classification of foods becomes another selective force to consider. One basis for classification is the ranking of foods in terms of their relative worth, from prestige or high-status foods to famine foods, or food for the poor. High-status prestige foods may be reserved for important people and occasions and are usually more expensive, more difficult to obtain, and associated with a dominant, powerful group. Roast animal meat is commonly a prestige food. Famine foods, reflecting financial stress or difficulties in obtaining food, are seldom served publicly. They are most often boiled so that less food is wasted. But they are not necessarily poor foods nutritionally. In fact, in Kenya, the greens, *sukuma wiki,* "to pull you through the week," are valuable sources of vitamins; but in Nairobi they are considered food for the poor.

Some food rankings are more complicated in origin. The shift in preference for white rice and white bread over brown rice and brown bread is harder to understand, since the latter products are of superior nutritional value. Yet white bread and white rice have been associated with high status for hundreds of years. Goody notes that in Europe when the feudal lord owned the mill, serfs tried to avoid having to pay for milling wheat and baking bread. Serfs and servants ate brown bread, while white bread made of highly milled white flour was served to the feudal lord. Similarly, milling rice was costly and could be avoided by cruder hand-milling in Asian households. Since the feudal lords controlled surplus rice, they benefited more from the improved storage capacity of milled white rice. Thus, control over the labor of others underlies the class distinctions symbolically associated with the more processed white bread and white rice (1982:231–232).

The evaluation of prestige and famine foods is strongly affected by the process of delocalization, the increased dependency on outside energy and resources in a community as a result of the modernization process. The shift to bottle feeding and infant formula is part of the process of delocalization of food resources facilitated by the perception of western foods as prestige goods. Coca-Cola is a clear example. Ritenbaugh points out that the rapid success of western foods in developing countries demonstrates not only the effectiveness of the manufacturers, but also "the willingness of people to alter food consumption patterns to gain status" (1978:118). When certain foods are evaluated as high or low prestige, people tend to choose foods that enhance their self-image. Cora du Bois also made this assumption explicit in her work in Alor, where she found that "if one can eat like the group he aspires towards, he has a right to identify with that group" (1941:655). On the other hand, Goody argues that the elite in Ghana prefer their traditional recipes and meal formats consisting of porridge and relish, even after extended contact with European-style foods. Here food recipes do not appear to be strongly differentiated by class (1982:177).

McGee refers to the process whereby countries become dependent on imported foods and foreign food patterns as "dietary colonialism" (1975:4). Such dependence often begins through colonial experiences where local groups desire foods initially consumed by an elite expatriate population. This pattern first affects the local elite and only later affects the wider population. At the same time, colonized groups may emulate the oppressor in developing their native foods.

In Kenya for example, canned milk products from England probably were adopted very quickly as prestige foods, since milk products were already part of the Kenyan diet. A middle-aged Kenyan professor recalled how the habit of drinking canned milk, which was brought in by the British to have with their tea, spread quickly among Kenyan workers. Once this milk became widespread in Kenyan society, it no longer marked elite status and became merely a popular drink. This raises the possibility that we should differentiate between items with clear cultural antecedents and those without such antecedents in explaining the creation of status symbols. Milk products in Kenya are less likely to remain as status symbols than milk products in non-dairying Thailand, for example. Similarly, objects like infant feeding bottles, which do not have clear cultural antecedents, may become status symbols because they are better vehicles for symbolic elaboration and allow for more varied interpretations than objects with clear cultural antecedents. Goody notes that some western-manufactured goods have so wide a distribution in African communities that they are no longer prestigious, valuable, or deluxe goods, but rather "commodities of mass commerce, staples of the local store and market" (1982:187).

Langdon (1975) in a study of the soap industry in Kenya describes this process as the inappropriate "taste transfer" from developed capitalist economies to developing countries, reflecting the colonial past of the country. Luxurious toilet soaps are better packaged, widely advertised, and more popular than their cheaper local counterparts. More serious consequences follow from taste preferences for less nutritious, more expensive western-style breakfast cereals in Kenya. Kaplinsky places the blame on costly promotion and advertising and the desire to consume prestige foods: "the consumption patterns of the expatriate elite are frequently copied by the nouveau riche Kenyans and are subsequently 'passed down' to the poor masses as standards worthy of emulation" (1981:231). As with breastmilk, the local, traditional cereal was vastly superior to the imported western substitute.

Manderson (1982) reviewed how bottle feeding with imported canned milk influenced Malaysian women. Nestlé and other companies began advertising condensed milk in the colonies as early as 1894, and encouraging its use for infant feeding. In the late 1920s, advertisements directed at the local elite began to appear in the Chinese and Malaysian press (1982:598). She is very clear about the efforts undertaken by the milk companies to change infant feeding habits: "they were competing for the market both of white women who in any case regarded breastfeeding as déclassé, if not downright animalistic, and indirectly of non-European elite women who were acutely sensitive to practices that might in any way distinguish them from their colonial rulers" (1982:605). Cicily Williams complained that in Singapore in the 1930s, "breastfeeding is not considered smart by a large section of the population, Chinese, Malay, European, Eurasian, Indian. . . . Among the well-to-do classes, the mother abandons breastfeeding because she wishes to be free to go out and play mahjong or because she considers it beneath her dignity to feed her own baby" (1986:66, 68).

The adoption of commercial infant foods in developing countries is part of this process of taste transfer, as food products become status symbols. While advocacy groups have documented this process for infant formula, the feeding bottles themselves have received less attention.

Chapter Five

Infant Feeding Bottles

Although feeding bottles are clearly implicated in the spread of breastmilk substitutes in third world countries, they are not discussed in detail in the regulations on the marketing of breastmilk substitutes and infant foods; nor have the manufacturers been required to put packaging messages on them about the superiority of breastfeeding. However, infant feeding bottles and teats are covered by the WHO/UNICEF Code of Marketing for Breastmilk Substitutes (1981). Article 5.4 states that no articles or utensils that might promote bottle feeding are to be distributed to pregnant women or mothers. But most regulations surrounding feeding bottles only monitor their technical standards and material quality. However, national regulations in some countries have gone much further than the WHO/UNICEF Code. The best known case of bottle regulation is the Baby Feed Supplies Control Bill of Papua New Guinea, passed in 1977. This act restricts the sale of feeding bottles, teats, and dummies unless authorized by medical personnel. Medical personnel are advised not to give this authorization unless it would be in the best interests of the infant and unless the infant's caretaker understands the instructions for their safe use. Critics of these regulations predicated a great increase in black-market sales of feeding bottles and the use of homemade bottle substitutes, but there have been few reports of such abuses and clear evidence for positive improvements in infant health (Biddulph 1980). Papua New Guinea is the only country to have legislated and enforced such comprehensive regulations for feeding bottles. A 1986 review of government legislation to support breastfeeding revealed that only three countries, Nicaragua, Tunisia, and Sri Lanka, reported legislation applied to utensils for bottle feeding (American Public Health Association 1986). Now that national codes modeled after the WHO/UNICEF Code are being developed, it is important to focus particular attention on feeding bottles as well as breastmilk substitutes for a number of reasons:

1. Some of the worst marketing and promotional abuses of the infant formula manufacturers—Nestlé in particular—have been corrected. For example, direct consumer advertising is all but ended; inappropriate labeling is in the process of being corrected; blatant techniques of sales promotion such as baby contests and milk nurses have been replaced with subtler forms of promotion through the medical profession.
2. Advertisements for feeding bottles and teats are common and unregulated in medical journals, newspapers, and popular magazines.
3. Although infant formula is almost always given through feeding bottles, they are used for a much wider range of products than infant formula and milk. In the urban areas covered in our four-country study, bottles often contained water, glucose solutions, fruit juices, rice water, tea, coffee, soda, starch paste, soups, and herbal tonics.
4. Feeding bottles, regardless of the quality of their contents, are damaging to lactation because they discourage infant sucking and contribute to nipple confusion in infants.
5. While infant formula may be too expensive for many households to purchase, feeding bottles can be acquired and used by even the poorest households. They can be purchased in urban markets for as little as twenty-five cents, although the more elaborate imported varieties may be quite expensive. They are a popular gift for a new baby. In poorer households, therefore, feeding bottles are probably distributed much more widely than infant formula. And if they are in the household, they will be used.

JOHN RYLANDS
UNIVERSITY
LIBRARY OF
MANCHESTER

6. Feeding bottles are more difficult to clean than a cup and spoon and are easily contaminated. Often, locally made bottles are harder to clean and sterilize than imported bottles if they are made with lower quality plastics.
7. If quality standards are not carefully enforced, feeding bottles may be dangerous. That is, they may be breakable, or have sharp edges and irregularities, or contain unacceptable levels of nitrosamines—a carcinogenic substance (see Craddock 1981).
8. Bottle feeding contributes to problems of tooth decay (bottle mouth syndrome) and malocclusion (poor "fit" between top and bottom teeth). Orthodontic correction of this condition is "nowhere more common than in America, where mass bottle feeding is of longest standing" (Minchin 1985:195).
9. Infant feeding bottles have wide-ranging synergistic effects. Their use may encourage poor care, such as leaving infants alone to "feed themselves," force-feeding by enlarging the feeding holes in the teat, and leaving young caretakers to watch or feed infants. Bottle feeding, by reducing body contact and infant stimulation, may have far-reaching effects on mother-infant interaction.

Feeding bottles require careful scrutiny and critical assessment to document their role in changing infant feeding patterns.

Bottles as Objects

Feeding bottles are common consumer goods in most developing countries. Using the levels of analysis proposed by Gottdiener (1985), we can consider feeding bottles as material objects with visible properties and functional objects with identifiable use value. However, feeding bottles can also be thought about, talked about, evaluated, displayed, traded, and exchanged. Here, the sign value of feeding bottles emerges.

From these different levels of analysis, it should be possible to determine how feeding bottles became status symbols.

Feeding bottles are currently one item among many small-scale consumer goods that can be found in elite supermarkets and open food markets throughout the third world, with the exception of countries like Papua New Guinea where they are not displayed for sale. Feeding bottles are not recent inventions; they have been identified from neolithic, late Bronze Age, and early Iron Age sites and in Roman burials from the first century A.D. Fildes documents a wide range of feeders made of horn, bone, pottery, glass, wood, leather, and metal. The European feeders were either round jug shapes, which gradually developed into sucking bottles, or the pap-boat, a feeder that was much easier to clean (1986:308). In 1841, Charles Windship of Massachusetts filed the first and last patent on a feeding container to be superimposed on a woman's breast to "induce the child to think it derives nourishment directly from the mother" (Drake 1948:509).

Regulations dealing with infant feeding bottles treat them as items of technology that must meet certain technical standards. These standards determine the quality of glass and plastic that are used, the acceptable amount of nitrosamines in the teat, the appropriateness of the teat shape, and the size of the feeding hole. The regulations also provide for quality control so that the bottles will not have sharp edges or irregularities. If manufacturers meet national standards, then the feeding bottles are considered acceptable. In any one community there will be both standard and substandard feeding bottles available, depending on how carefully technical standards are monitored and enforced. In many countries the inspection of imported and locally made feeding bottles is not a high priority.

A more serious problem for the international manufacturers, is counterfeited feeding bottles. These bottles display a prestigious trade mark, such as NUK or CHICCO, but are made locally and are of poorer quality. This counterfeiting reduces the market for expensive imported bottles and makes regulation even more difficult. Only a discerning shopper can tell a genuine CHICCO bottle from a counterfeit one selling at a lower price.

Feeding bottles are only part of the system of specialized infant consumer goods often advertised and sold together, and their meaning is derived from their place in sets or series of objects. Special chairs, cribs, and other baby furniture are increasingly available in urban centers. Poor rural and urban households may not be able to purchase most infant consumer goods, but they can afford cheap feeding bottles.

Much of this equipment encourages the distancing of mother and infant. At the same time, this distancing increases a mother's control over her own life and that of her infant. The elaborate equipment associated and advertised with bottle feeding includes sterilizer sets, tongs, cleaning brushes and solutions, various carrying cases, thermos bottles with nipple tops, and an increasingly large number of different kinds of bottles. In October of 1982, the following products associated with bottle feeding were available in the dry goods section of a Nairobi supermarket:

1. An electric bottle warmer with a bottle inside. (393 K.Sh., U.S. $51.09)
2. A small bottle with a screw-on feeding spoon for "introducing baby to weaning foods successfully" (i.e., earlier). When the bottle is tipped up, the contents flow into the spoon. (32.50 K.Sh., U.S. $4.22)
3. A small 150 cc plastic bottle with a screw-on attachment to convert it into baby's first drinking cup, "to accustom baby to a cup." Included in the package was a nipple with extra-small holes for a premature baby. (32.50 K.Sh., U.S. $4.22)

4. A bright orange quilted carrier with a special thermos to hold hot water and a separate container to hold the right amount of infant formula, "so that there is no danger of spoiled milk." (140 K.Sh., U.S. $18.20)
5. A 250 cc CHICCO Pyrex bottle. (47.50 K.Sh., U.S. $6.17)
6. Cannon smooth-necked feeder (250 cc) with a special neck so that milk will not stick in the crevices (imported from England). (24 K.Sh., U.S. $3.12)
7. Nursery Griptight Freeflo Feeder with a special nipple to avoid colic. It is shaped so that is "easy for baby to hold." (13.20 K.Sh., U.S. $1.72)
8. Thermos with a screw-in nipple "to keep babies' milk warm all day." (CHICCO 290 K.Sh., U.S. $37.70)
9. Bottle with a screw-on handle so that babies can hold the bottle themselves. (CHICCO 47.50 K.Sh., U.S. $6.17)
10. Kiddy Freeflo Feeder (150 cc) made by Sumaria Industries, Nairobi. (11.95 K.Sh., U.S. $1.55)
11. Teats. (2.50 K.Sh., U.S. $.32)

Other associated products include Maws and Milton solutions for purifying water so that it is not necessary to boil the bottles to clean them. The products are sold in chemists' shops: Maws solution, 56 tablets for 49.85 K.Sh. (U.S. $6.48); Milton solution, 600 ml for 25 K.Sh. (U.S. $3.25).

When these prices were recorded, 8 Kenya shillings were worth U.S. $1.05; for comparison, the maternity fee for delivery at the National Hospital was 60 K.Sh., and housemaids earned around 300 K.Sh. per month. Feeding bottles and related infant equipment are rapidly becoming necessities that reflect and deflect maternal commitment and love.

Instrumental Value of Feeding Bottles

Infant feeding bottles are obviously useful to mothers and infant caretakers; otherwise they would not be so widely used

TABLE 5.1
Bottle Feeding at Three Months

	Number	*Breastmilk Substitutes in Bottle*	*Exclusive Bottle Feeding*
		(Percent)	(Percent)
Nairobi	50	65	2
Bangkok	113	55	43
Semarang	61	20	18
Bogotá	26	63	31

in many parts of the world. In the infant feeding practices study, feeding bottles used in all four countries contained breastmilk substitutes, other liquids, and food mixtures. Table 5.1 shows the percentages of women who used bottles for breastmilk substitutes either for mixed feeding or exclusive bottle feeding their three-month-old infants. From these figures, we can see that bottle feeding was common among these women, although exclusive bottle feeding is less common. Cup and spoon feeding is quite rare, although it is occasionally used.

In descriptions of infant feeding patterns, it is often assumed that the phrase, "bottle fed infant," refers to exclusive bottle feeding from birth. More recently, attention has focused on the "triple-nipple" pattern of mixed feeding (Latham et al. 1986). But bottle feeding fits into infant feeding patterns in a variety of different ways. Below are listed some patterns of use abstracted from ethnographic observations in the four-country study:

1. Exclusive Bottle. Instead of initiating breastfeeding, a small proportion of mothers from wealthier households fed their infants breastmilk substitutes from bottles

from birth. In some of the ethnographic cases, parents bottle fed an adopted child with a feeding bottle.

2. Newborn Bottle. Some infants were bottle fed for the first three days after birth. They were generally given glucose mixtures or infant formula for their first feeds. The newborn bottle is particularly common when mothers give birth in hospitals and in areas where colostrum is devalued (particularly Indonesia).
3. Top-up Bottle. The top-up bottle was used in all four sites to supplement breastfeeding or "top-up" the feed. Most top-up bottles contained infant formula or milk and were given immediately after breastfeeding. Often the regular top-up bottle resulted in insufficient milk by causing the production of breastmilk to decline. The top-up bottle can thus contribute to the early termination of breastfeeding.
4. Regular Substitute Bottle. The regular substitute bottle replaces one or more breastfeedings, often in the middle of the day. It is quite common for women employed some distance from home to use a regular substitute bottle; this usually contains a milk-based breastmilk substitute.
5. Temporary Substitute Bottle. The temporary substitute bottle replaces all breastfeeding for a brief time. This occurs when the mother or baby is sick and she fears her milk might affect the baby, or when a mother has to leave her infant for three or four days. This pattern may result in insufficient milk if the mother does not express her breastmilk or anticipate the need to build up her milk supply on her return.
6. Public Feeding Bottle. In all four countries, some mothers felt that breastfeeding in public was inappropriate and carried a feeding bottle with them for feeding during church services, clinic visits, meetings, or parties.

The rest of the time, these mothers breastfed in the privacy of their homes.

7. Sleep Bottle. Occasionally, mothers who otherwise breastfed their infants gave them a bottle to take to bed with them so that they could sleep undisturbed.
8. Comfort Bottle. Similarly, a comfort bottle might be given to a child as a pacifier. In Thailand, the plastic pacifiers were unpopular. Mothers felt they cheated babies by encouraging them to suck without getting anything to drink. Occasionally, these comfort bottles were given empty.
9. Weaning Food Bottle. The weaning food bottle is probably a recent innovation that was encouraged by the marketing of special feeding bottles with large holes or beaker spouts for this purpose and by the promotion of commercial weaning foods like Cerelac. These bottles can be particularly dangerous since an infant can easily be force-fed in this manner. They also encourage the earlier introduction of weaning foods. Finally, weaning foods may be overdiluted with water to allow them to flow more easily through bottles with small holes not designed for weaning foods.
10. Medicine Bottle. Bottles are strongly favored for giving infants both western-style patent medicines and herbal mixtures. Medicines in powdered form are dissolved in liquids and fed from feeding bottles. Mothers in Bogotá gave their infants a total of 179 different herbal mixtures in feeding bottles (such as sugar water, cinnamon, and broth). These combinations, often mixed with vegetable water or soup to which some additional milk powder had been added, were prepared individually for infants or children to adjust their dietary intake to suit their needs and improve their health.

11. Water Bottle. Mothers often felt their infants needed a drink of water from a bottle because they were "thirsty" even after breastfeeding.

These patterns give an indication of the complexity of the activity of bottle feeding. It is likely that each pattern of use has different determinants and consequences. For example, the top-up bottle and the temporary substitute bottle may contribute more to insufficient milk than the regular substitute bottle. The weaning food bottle may have more negative consequences for infant health than the public feeding bottle. Feeding bottles are becoming increasingly popular for weaning foods in developing countries. Encouraged by the elaboration of infant feeders, teats with large holes, and special beaker lips to screw on to feeding bottles, mothers in all four cities are able to find a number of indigenous and commercial weaning foods to serve in feeding bottles. These products range from flour mixtures to "thicken" a bottle to porridges such as *uji* in Kenya. In all four sites, commercial cereals are available and popular, particularly among higher-income women. In the poor urban households, feeding bottles are well entrenched in the strategies mothers develop to solve problems of infant care. No maternal and child health program is likely to succeed in decreasing the use of feeding bottles until the programs understand what problems feeding bottles solve for women and then suggest alternative solutions.

Bottle as Symbol

Feeding bottles are not simply used to feed infants: they are also used as part of a broader semiotic or sign system to communicate something about the user. Goods acquire "meaning in use" beyond their instrumental value. Advertisers are well aware of these meanings and build on them to increase the appeal of their products.

Objects like feeding bottles are suitable for symbolic elaboration because they are convenient, visible markers of status and identity. Mary Douglas's significant book, *World of Goods* (1979), argues that consumers' choices of purchased goods are attempts to impose identity and meaning on their environments. For the poorest consumers who have few opportunities for establishing their identity, the acquisition and display of small-scale consumer goods may be one of the few means they have to communicate how they expect to be treated. For the poor in Thailand, for example, these symbols of development and modernization offer stability, serve as mechanisms of status attribution, and create the image that they have some control over their lives (Meesook 1978:112).

How do goods like feeding bottles acquire expanded symbolic meanings? First, people are likely to purchase brands that enhance their self-image. Semarang mothers, for example, were quite explicit about the kinds of people who buy CHICCO bottles and very conscious of their higher price. Mothers may simply desire to own an easily achievable status symbol to enhance their own self-image. Second, some mothers wanted to emulate high-status women. Rosa, Amporn, and Grace, who worked as housemaids, learned some of their approaches to infant feeding from their employers. The social value of feeding bottles is also increased by their association with valued institutions like hospitals. Hospitals in all four countries use feeding bottles rather than a cup and spoon for giving glucose and other feeds to newborns.

Just as the picture of a feeding bottle containing a marasmic infant has been a powerful symbol for the activists seeking to limit the promotion of infant formula in developing countries, so the feeding bottle for many women in the third world is a symbol of their freedom from worry about the quality and quantity of their breastmilk. Mothers like Amporn may not link the increased morbidity associated with bottle feeding to the bottle, but to the contents, thereby initiating a constant experimental testing of new kinds of breastmilk substitutes.

The symbolic significance or sign value of feeding bottles arises out of the ordinary or literal meanings of the bottle as antecedent object. That is, certain qualities of feeding bottles make them suitable vehicles for symbolic elaboration. The objects themselves are associated with food and feeding, already an emotionally charged domain; they are small, yet reasonably complex (that is composed of more than one part); although they are created for a special purpose, they are made to resemble something else (initially, a human breast and nipple—currently, Fred Flintstone); they come in a wide range of prices, from very cheap to expensive; they are usually transparent so that user and observer can see the substance inside.

The symbolic significance of bottles arises both from the literal meaning of the feeding bottle and the context of its use. The way individuals assign meaning to these objects depends on their individual experience. However, individual experience with feeding bottles would not in itself be sufficient to create a status symbol. It is the advertising copy and the promotional messages that made explicit the symbolic connections that are only suggested through individual experience. Over time, individual interpretations of this object have been made to overlap significantly through repetitive associations of feeding bottles with the concepts of wealth, health, science, and modernity. The bottle emerges as a status symbol through the intersection of individual meanings and advertising claims.

The following observations are based on an examination of thirty advertisements for feeding bottles and infant formula (if a feeding bottle figures prominently in the ad) appearing in popular and medical magazines. They span the years from

TABLE 5.2
Distribution of advertisements

	North America and Europe	*Asia, Africa, Latin America*
Pre 1920s	2	—
1930s	3	—
1940s	0	1
1950s	3	—
1960s	6	—
1970s	1	2
1980s	1	11

1910 to 1983 and come from North America, Europe, Latin America, Africa, and South and Southeast Asia (see Table 5.2).

Wealth is not emphasized in the direct copy in the ads in European or developing countries. Rather, the low cost of the bottle is stressed. However, wealth is the context within which bottle feeding activities take place. Well-dressed mothers and infants in modern homes frame the activity of bottle feeding. The plump healthy babies are themselves indirect symbols of wealth.

Modernity is stressed in direct copy by such phrases as: "latest advance in modern technology"; "new, modern, deluxe"; "a break with tradition". Much more significant both in direct copy and visual presentation is the evocation of science. References are both direct and indirect through association with the medical profession. Direct references include: "product of long years of scientific development"; "orthodontic nipple"; "timed to feed at the correct rate"; "scientifically designed." Visual cues are even more effective in creating this image. Results of experiments comparing different methods of sterilizing bottles, scientific publications stuffed into feeding bottles, and laboratory scenes are used as background for the copy.

Medical personnel are shown using feeding bottles, and the copy stresses the recommendations of pediatricians and doctors. Testimonials of qualified medical experts or authorities who recommend use of particular products were especially popular in North American ads between 1930 and 1940 (Leiss, Kline, and Jhally 1986:120). Photographs of feeding bottles used by nurses underscore the health benefits of specific brands of bottles and nipples, such as anticolic nipples or bottles that prevent diarrhea and other digestive disorders. The direct copy refers to their use in approved hospital procedures and emphasizes the invariant, dependable qualities of the bottles and nipples, as well as the contents of the bottle. This image is reinforced not only by pictures of measuring cups and spoons but also by prominent displays of the numbers on the side of the feeding bottles. In summary, these ads emphasize science, with wealth and modernity as background context. However, the three themes fit well together as a complex; wealth-science-modernity.

The secondary meaning of feeding bottles is seen most clearly when bottle feeding is compared with breastfeeding. In the ads of both developed and developing countries, the symbolic meaning of feeding bottles is emphasized through direct and implicit contrasts with breastfeeding. Western ads favor charts comparing the protein, fat, and carbohydrate content of mother's milk and alternative artificial feeds such as infant formula or evaporated milk. Other ads stress the fact that bottle feeding duplicates the desirable qualities of breastfeeding. A 1981 ad from Brazil featured a close-up photograph of a woman's body from neck to waist, with breasts exposed. This photograph was contrasted with pictures of packages of sealed feeding bottles and women modestly feeding their infants with bottles. Although the copy draws attention to the alleged similarity between maternal nipple and rubber teat, the underlying message of exposure vs. modesty is much more striking. A similar contrast is made explicit in an ad showing mothers breastfeeding at home and bottle feeding in a doctor's office.

Bottles figure prominently in ads promoting mixed feeding strategies for breastfeeding mothers. In this context, feeding bottles are presented as objects that assist natural breastfeeding, as a "bridge to successful nursing. . . ." For a mother uncertain as to how she should feed her baby, bottles are presented as aids that allow her to get a good night's sleep, to feed her infant in public without embarrassment, and to have time off for recreation with her husband. The feeding bottle represents the mother's control over her infant's development and daily routine, and over her own personal time. Advertisements for bottles, building on mothers' fears of insufficient milk, lactation failure, or the ultimate fear of infant death suggest that bottles provide mothers with a means of controlling their infants' health. Certain bottles and nipples claim to protect the baby's health. A Philippine ad for Evenflo nipples (1981) explained how mothers can enlarge the hole in the nipple so that the baby will not get tired sucking, and how the structure of the nipple lessens the chances of colic. An Indian ad suggests that mothers can hand down their polycarbonate Babycare bottle from baby to baby, as if the manufacturer recognized that the feeding bottle may be a status symbol in some households. They further this connection in the copy: "For their children's health and safety, mothers abroad rely on an alternative which is totally safe. Now you can too" (from *Femina* magazine, Feb. 23, 1980: 32).

In sum, ads for bottles claim that feeding bottles save mother's precious time, are convenient, and easy to fill. Moreover, the ads often feature the baby holding the bottle with its hands (or feet as in one Indian ad). Feeding bottles appear to give mothers more control over their own lives and the lives of their infants.

Role of Advertising

Borgoltz, in his report, "Economic and Business Aspects of Infant Formula Promotion," submitted to UNICEF and WHO (1979), argues that the development of brand image is important in transforming infant formula, a functional product, into a status or prestige product. This is done by developing an image involving the ego or self-image of the mother that connotes membership in a "higher" social group. This is especially true in developing countries where infant formula use and bottle feeding are associated with modernized elites (Borgoltz 1979:19,25). This is not to claim that advertising alone creates the symbolic value of bottle feeding. Rather, advertising uses existing associations to build these second-order meanings of wealth, science, and modernity. Certainly, direct consumer advertising of infant formula was only a part of a much more complex marketing strategy, including competitive pricing and promotion through health services.

How potent is advertising? Industry supporters tend to minimize the role of advertising, often arguing that there is no scientific proof that advertising affects infant feeding methods. Mary Douglas dismisses "theories of consumption which assume a puppet consumer, prey to the advertiser's wiles" as "frivolous, even dangerous" (1979:89). "Mothers in Poverty," published as Vol. 2 No. 3 of the *Lactation Review* (1977), summarizes and comments on papers presented at the International Conference on Human Lactation held in New York in 1977. McCollough, a third world research specialist at Ross Laboratories, presented the industry's viewpoint on the impact of infant formula in developing nations. The *Lactation Review* comments on his presentation: "McCollough reminds us that the USSR with a high level of modernization and no advertising has just contracted for a huge infant formula manufacturing plant. Advertising techniques of the multinational corporations probably exacerbate an already existing problem, but to credit them with superhuman influence and power is to put down the intelligence and humanity of the mothers" (Human Lactation Center 1977:8). Activists are generally accused by industry supporters of assuming that third world women are dumb or brainwashed by advertising. This is certainly not the issue, as Campbell points out: "Critics do not focus on the intellectual capabilities of Third World mothers but rather on the economic realities of their existence" (1984:550). On the other hand, serious ethical questions arise when advertising is directed to consumers less experienced in the analysis of advertising.

A leading market researcher provides a similar comment on how the public views advertising research: "The popular press sees it [advertising research] as a malodorous device to hoodwink a gullible public, corrupt morals, and induce unsuspecting consumers into squandering their rent money on hair sprays and junk food because it gives advertisers the wherewithal to transmit their sales messages directly to the brain's control center, bypassing Reason's protective shield, and to harvest irrational wants and needs below the level of conscious awareness . . . most researchers would be thrilled to find their advertising research had one-tenth this power" (Haller 1983:58).

The facts that the infant formula industry spends millions per year on advertising and is steadily increasing its sales in the third world suggest that a less naive view of advertising is called for. A neoliberal and Marxist critique of advertising takes a very different position, arguing that the function of national consumer product advertising" was, and still is to create demand among consumers to ensure that the goods produced in such large numbers by mass production are bought in equally large numbers, so that the owners of the factories producing them can secure adequate returns on their investments. To this end, advertising is a manipulative tool, controlling the market by creating false needs in consumers, and by extolling a general ethos of consumption whereby all needs come to be fulfilled through the purchase of goods in the marketplace" (Leiss, Klein, and Jhally 1986:16).

Bottle Feeding as Technology Transfer

In the chapter on medicalization, we reviewed how the transfer of health technology to developing countries encouraged the growth of hospital-based curative medicine and created a market for the products of western biotechnology and pharmaceutical companies. Many of these health technology transfers could be considered inappropriate. Rarely is any consideration given to the implications of the technology transfer for women. Birth control products are an excellent example of a transfer where the costs for women were not fully calculated. Feeding bottles, a form of simple technology, are assumed to facilitate the task of infant feeding. By subjecting feeding bottles to the same kind of analysis proposed for larger technology transfers, these assumptions can be tested.

New items of technology such as feeding bottles require new patterns of behavior for their appropriate use. Although feeding bottles are not new inventions, their widespread use throughout the developing world is relatively recent. The bottles, which were developed in Europe and North America, are now easily accessible in the developing world, both in urban supermarkets and tiny kiosks in remote rural areas. Although this is an example of the transfer of extremely simple technology, Cappon's warning is still appropriate: "skipping links in the technological chain does not allow for the required time for absorption of the concomitant ideology" (1971:9). When goods are transferred from one society or one context to another, the skills and experience for using them are not always transferred with them. The adaptive strategy for using goods successfully may be lost in the transfer.

In his classic study of steel axes for Stone Age Australians, Sharp (1952) illustrates how a change in one item of technology can have significant effects in a number of seemingly unconnected domains such as religion, trade, and even gender ideology. So, too, infant feeding bottles involve substantial changes in both knowledge and household activity patterns.

In spite of a decade of intensive examination of breastfeeding and bottle feeding during the infant formula controversy, we still have very little knowledge of how bottle feeding technology is transferred to developing countries and how it facilitates infant care. The framework for technology transfer developed by Mary Anderson (1985) raises questions about how new technology affects the doer, location, and timing of the activity, and the skills and knowledge necessary for carrying out the new activity.

1. Does technology transfer affect the doer of the activity? It would be easy to assume, as advertisements for infant formula and feeding bottles suggest, that bottle feeding frees women to perform more rewarding and lucrative tasks. This is certainly not always the case in rural areas where breastfeeding is more easily combined with other farm tasks than are bottle preparation and feeding. In the urban situation, what is the impact of bottle feeding on the sexual division of labor? Does bottle

feeding alter the role assignment of the task? In Nairobi, 84 percent of mothers giving milk to their infants and 82 percent of mothers giving infant formula bottle feed their infants themselves. In Semarang, mothers generally prepare the infant formula themselves, even if a grandmother gives it to the infant. Of those mothers not breastfeeding, 42 percent bottle feed their infant themselves.

In Indonesia and Kenya, it is clear that fathers or other adult males rarely relieved mothers of this task. In both countries, about 10 percent of mothers using breastmilk substitutes hired a maid who did the feeding, thus freeing them for other activities, including social events, in addition to formal work. Other family members such as grandmothers or young daughters may take over bottle feeding, but in our study, mothers generally remained responsible for bottle feeding their infants.

As new technologies move into an area, the ability to handle them is usually associated with relatively high status (Anderson 1985:61). High-income women delighted in showing their expensive imported equipment and cleaning solutions for the upkeep of feeding bottles. But there is no evidence that men's occasional use of feeding bottles confers any higher status on bottle feeding, since infant feeding is still considered women's work.

2. Does technology transfer affect the location of the activity? New technologies may alter the location of the productive activity. Breastfeeding can be done anywhere mother and infant are together. If bottles are prepared hygenically, then bottle feeding may restrict the location of infant feeding. In practice, bottle feeding is preferred in public places. In Nairobi, 77 percent of mothers agreed that it is better to bottle feed a baby in a public place such as a clinic or church. The adoption of bottle feeding technology does not necessarily alter the location of the activity of infant feeding, since feeding bottles are generally prepared ahead of time and carried around like portable breasts.

3. Does technology transfer affect the timing of the activity? There is little agreement in the infant feeding literature about whether breastfeeding or bottle feeding takes more of a woman's time. In the urban four-country study, women had a wide range of attitudes about the time spent feeding infants. About half (47 percent) of the Bangkok mothers surveyed found breastfeeding inconvenient and time-consuming, 33 percent agreed that breastmilk substitutes were less trouble than breastfeeding. For these women, there are many other activities competing for their time. Both formal and informal work may require substantial transportation time. More significantly, the time spent breastfeeding is not considered enjoyable time. If time spent in other ways can be both more enjoyable and more profitable, breastfeeding will not fare well.

In contrast, most Semarang mothers (88 percent) disagreed with the statement that bottle feeding is less messy and troublesome than breastfeeding; nor did they use shortage of time or inconvenience as a reason for beginning supplementary feeding or terminating breastfeeding. These women do not take the option of not breastfeeding very seriously and thus arrange their activities around breastfeeding.

Similarly, in Nairobi, breastfeeding is taken for granted, although 60 percent of mothers surveyed agree that bottle feeding is the fastest way to feed an infant, particularly in comparison with cup and spoon. But few Nairobi mothers were greatly pressed for time since work opportunities were minimal for the poorest women.

In Colombia, ethnographic evidence suggests that women do not idealize the convenient, fast way to feed an infant. Rather, mothers emphasized the time they spent on preparing complex food mixtures for their children, as if more time spent equated with greater care and love. The more elaborate and time-consuming homemade infant food recipes were considered better for infants, and more dependable.

Bottle feeding requires more preparation time, particularly for poor women without labor-saving devices. Time is needed for obtaining fuel if needed, obtaining and boiling water, preparing the mixture, and cleaning the bottles and equipment after feeding. Feeding cannot be a spontaneous response to an infant's cry but must minimally be planned to allow for preparation time. If women are both breastfeeding and bottle feeding, their time spent in infant feeding doubles, a fact that encourages Bangkok mothers in particular to cease breastfeeding after they have established a bottle feeding routine.

Bottle feeding may "save more time" when it is used for weaning foods. These foods are diluted, combined with breastmilk substitutes, and served in a bottle.

With special bottles and teats, a mother can get solids into an infant before the infant is old enough to be spoon fed. An Indian consumer group has had some feeders banned, since infants choke easily when force-fed by pushing on the vacuum disc to speed the ingestion of food. The negative health consequences from early complementary solids or from forced feeding, however, may cost a mother much more time in caring for a sick infant.

However, when women bottle feed a young infant instead of breastfeeding, the scheduling and periodicity of the task do not change greatly. That is, the task of infant feeding is a high-periodicity (high-frequency), nonpostponable, menial task, which accounts for its low value and subsequent assignment to low-rank individuals, according to Mary Douglas (1979:119–124). Infant feeding is an intensive task, accomplished in brief bursts of activity several times during the day. Breastfeeding, in particular, is compatible with other high-frequency household tasks, and a feature of most women's domestic work patterns is the accomplishment of several high-periodicity tasks simultaneously.

4. Does technology transfer affect the skills and knowledge necessary for the new activity? Breastfeeding and bottle feeding, or breastmilk and infant formula, are often falsely equated in the minds of many health professionals and consumers in both developed and developing countries. Consequently, mothers do not anticipate problems as they begin using bottles for feeding their infants. However, there are certain skills and knowledge that should be acquired along with the technology of bottle feeding.

Ideally, mothers need to accept the germ theory of disease causation in order to spend the extra time and money necessary for sterilizing bottles and storing leftover breastmilk substitutes appropriately. A mother's past experience and knowledge of breastfeeding an infant are not necessarily sufficient for successful bottle feeding. The mechanical patterns of sucking milk are quite different in breastfeeding and bottle feeding. During breastfeeding, an infant's mouth is wide open and milk is extracted through the action of the infant's tongue and jaw. During bottle feeding, an infant closes its mouth around the teat (its jaws do not need to compress the nipple to extract the fluid) and uses its tongue to slow down the flow of fluid to keep from gagging (Minchin 1985:90). Infants who try to breastfeed in this manner may become frustrated due to nipple confusion. Caretakers who use feeding bottles may need some instruction on correct techniques for bottle feeding, particularly if they are using bottles with cheap, poorly formed teats.

Additionally, new patterns of infant handling are necessary to alleviate the problem of swallowed air, which is much more common in bottle fed babies than breastfed babies. While western breastfeeding manuals mention burping the baby, they stress that this is rarely needed in breastfed babies, except for the "gulpers" who may try to nurse too fast and swallow some air. However, burping a baby is not a common part of infant care in nonwestern societies where the infant care model is a breastfed baby. Bottle fed infants easily ingest air and require mechanical means to remove the air. These techniques may not be part of the infant care repertoire in many societies. Failure to burp an infant may result in stomach upsets, which caretakers often attempt to relieve by the use of readily available patent medicines.

Finally, the stools of breastfed infants are infrequent, soft, and formless in contrast to the harder, larger, more frequent stools of infants fed cow's milk, infant formula, or other foods. Caretakers used to breastfed babies may be surprised and concerned by the difference and respond inappropriately to the stools of an infant fed with formula. The ethnographic accounts describe women who treat their bottle fed infants with stool softeners, laxatives, and suppositories in an attempt to regulate their infants. The problem of constipation for bottle fed babies is not new. In Malaysia (1925), Baby's Own Tablets were advertised to deal with fever, bowel irregularities, digestive problems, diarrhea, colic, etc., "but also specifically for bottle fed infants who, according to the advertisements 'most often need help' to avoid constipation" (Manderson 1982:603).

The skills for caring for a breastfed baby can be transferred from mother to daughter or acquired from a support group of experienced breastfeeding mothers, as is the case in many western societies. The skills necessary for correct bottle feeding are acquired from medical personnel and infant formula manufacturers who provide books, pamphlets, demonstrations, and posters to clinics and directly to mothers wherever possible. Local advertising may fail to provide the necessary information about bottle feeding and breastmilk substitutes and instead provide an image of the user as a modern western consumer.

It is this dependence on the manufacturers to provide the educational material and information necessary for appropriate use of the new technology that is at the heart of the breast-bottle controversy. On the one hand, the transfer of bottle technology requires the acquisition of new skills; on the other hand, the "education" becomes effective promotion for the transfer of technology that is, in many cases, inappropriate and dangerous.

CHAPTER SIX

The Pattern That Connects

IN THE LAST FOUR CHAPTERS, we have examined a number of submerged discourses about breastfeeding and the breast-bottle controversy and offered some explanations about how they became submerged. In doing this, each perspective was examined somewhat in isolation. But breastfeeding is part of a complex system that interacts with many facets of the environment. We cannot begin to unravel the complexities of infant feeding by examining only one part of the system—urban environments, empowerment of women, medicalization of infant feeding, or the commoditization of food. In fact, tinkering with only one part of the system, such as hospital-based promotion of breastfeeding or provision of high-protein weaning foods, may have unintended consequences for the whole system. We have also seen that neither understanding of these system linkages nor scientific knowledge about any or all of the components necessarily leads to social action or policy initiatives to suppoort breastfeeding.

The breast-bottle controversy serves as a constant reminder

of the connections between environmental conditions, empowerment of women, medicalization of life, and the commoditization of food. The issue is deeply embedded in these interlocking systems. This argument can be illustrated using the example of environmental pollutants and breastmilk, an example that shows how infant feeding is linked to broader environmental concerns. But it is also a reminder that advocacy discourse must intervene to question how to interpret environmental effects on infant feeding choices from the broader perspective of sustainable development.

Breastfeeding and Environmental Pollution

Every day there are claims made about some environmental pollutant's effect on breastmilk—regardless of whether the causal mechanism is identified. In many ways, breastfeeding rates and lactation performance act as a gauge for judging when our capacity to adapt to environmental stresses—air, water, and noise pollution, toxins, radiation—has been overstrained. Breastfeeding becomes a mirror that reflects how well nations are meeting women's needs, and maternal health becomes a primary measure of the sustainability and quality of life. For regardless of what research determines to be safe levels of pollutants in human milk and the assessment of the long-term risks, it is generally true that breastmilk production is a concentrator of what is in the environment of the mother. Thus, any policies directed at promoting breastfeeding also create pressures for environmental safeguards.

From the perspective of environmental health, researchers have documented how and why environmental pollution may affect the safety of breastfeeding. For example, some fat-soluble and water-insoluble organochlorines and bromides such as polychlorinated biphenyls (PCB's), pesticides, and DDT may concentrate in breastmilk (Rall 1979:233). Rall states that breastmilk contains up to 300 times the concentration of PCB's found in whole blood (1979:234). The concentration of PCB's in the environment used to be the result of sporadic leaks or mistakes, but now it should be viewed as general environmental contamination. Pregnant and lactating women are advised to avoid eating freshwater fish from contaminated waters (Rall 1979:237). While lactating women can regulate their own intake of pollutants ingested through food to some extent, they have little control over the pollutants entering infant formula. As Minchin notes, "to sensationalize the problems of, say, pesticides in human milk is much easier than to document the chemical contamination of infant formula—or attempting to halt the pollution at its source" (1985:247).

A number of advocacy groups concerned with infant and maternal health voiced fears about the possibility of breastmilk contamination from the Chernobyl accident. Medical advice to mothers under conditions of contamination from radiation is to reduce their own intake of cow's milk and keep breastfeeding (Haschke et al. 1987:410). In response to fears about radiation contamination in infant formula, Dumex in Malaysia launched a vigorous advertising campaign emphasizing that all their infant food products were made from uncontaminated New Zealand milk. Overall, breastfeeding advocates stress that the known benefits of breastmilk outweigh the unknown possible hazards from pollutants in breastmilk. By focusing on individual solutions, such as advising breastfeeding mothers not to eat contaminated fish, we may neglect the more general and long-term strategy of pressuring industry to stop contaminating the fish in the first place. But while breastmilk appears to be one means of introducing PCB's to infants, breastmilk production is one of the only known mechanisms for the excretion of PCB's from the mother's body—another example of the complex symbiotic interaction between maternal and infant environments. But studies on the health consequences of pollutants are difficult to evaluate. *Pediatrics,* for example, published an assessment of the scientific evidence relating to infant feeding, which was funded by Ross Laboratories, manufacturers of Similac and other infant formulas. Minchin points out that in the report, "while the hazards of chemicals in breast milk were clearly delineated, there was no mention at all of chemical pollution of formula. Yet we know that the pasture, the feed, the milk, the tanker that transports it, the water used in manufacture and preparation, the cans that store it, not only are at risk but actually have been seriously contaminated in the past" (1985:26). The research discourse often contains what appear to be blatant contradictions in research results between those with evidence to show that synthetic chemical pesticides are a proven health hazard and those who hold an opposing view (Benarde 1973:110). More significantly, the World Commission on Environment and Development reports that "no toxicity data exists for nearly 80 per cent of the chemicals used in commercial products and processes inventoried under the Toxic Substances Control Act" (1987:224). This underscores the importance of political will and advocacy action in order to make difficult trade-offs.

Fear of breastmilk contamination itself could also be a major cause of lactation failure. Concerns about the effects of radiation and AIDS on breastmilk are well publicized. For example, in an editorial in the *Wall Street Journal* (June 19, 1986), Adelman casually mentions the difficulty breastmilk banks in developing countries face when they have to manage the pasturization of breastmilk necessary to kill the AIDS virus in breastmilk. Although there has been only one documented case of a child getting AIDS from her infected mother's breastmilk, mothers infected with AIDS have been advised not to breastfeed. However, a WHO meeting in Geneva concluded that breastmilk is the safest form of nourishment for most infants, even when the mother is infected. The uncertainties concerning AIDS could lead to panic and to the closing of breastmilk banks. A long-term strategy might be to investigate the role of breastfeeding in strengthening the immune system.

Breastfeeding and even infant feeding are easily dismissed as trivial, narrow topics compared with other more pressing development issues. Yet a full systems analysis of the implications arising from policies to increase breastfeeding indicates how broad the ramifications could be. But, as with many other development issues, we cannot expect to see or measure changes after a year. The changes envisioned are long-term changes in the way people think about themselves and their relations with their children. As people begin to identify the institutions and relations that interfere with breastfeeding, they may recognize parallels with other problems related to pesticides, health care systems, food and drug companies, or their work environments. Empowering women in developed and developing countries to recognize their interconnectedness with these broad issues becomes a consciousness-raising experience that is both immediate and personal.

Past policy initiatives at UNICEF have stressed breastfeeding promotion. Breastfeeding policies can be linked to other infant health campaigns such as immunization, where breastfeeding provides the first immunizing experience; family planning, where breastfeeding is more effective than all other forms of contraception combined; growth monitoring, where lack of breastmilk in the second year of life contributes to a significant energy deficit; and to oral rehydration therapy. The latter is an effective therapy, but without a simultaneous increase in breastfeeding, the incidence of diarrhea is unlikely to decrease. Promotion of oral rehydration therapy in isolation may also reinforce faulty ideas about the value of glucose feeds as a "cure" for diarrhea.

But immunization, family planning, growth monitoring, and oral rehydration therapy, all provide opportunities for pharmaceutical companies to make large, profitable contracts with governments, aid agencies, and multilateral organizations. These campaigns are more deeply entrenched in the development industry than are breastfeeding promotion campaigns. This is reflected in the 1987 UNICEF report on the state of the world's children, which stresses immunization, growth monitoring, and oral rehydration, and places little emphasis on breastfeeding.

ERRORS IN THINKING

It is, of course, easier to try to change people's attitudes toward infant feeding through education or by changing hospital routines than to demand broad environmental changes in living conditions and the redistribution of power and resources. But the World Commission on Environment and Development argued that "the distribution of power and influence within society lies at the heart of most environment and development challenges" (1987:38). Bateson argues that environmental problems stem from three root causes: technological progress, population increase, and errors in thinking (1972:490). Ideas that humans control the environment, that misery is part of the human condition, that the problems are too mammoth to justify any reform initiatives, and that technology will solve human problems are serious obstacles to improving environmental conditions. Bateson recognizes the powerful barrier of vested interests that block environmental reforms and make it difficult to see the pattern that connects.

Errors in thinking are difficult to document and certainly difficult to link directly to actions and decisions affecting the world system. But suppose Bateson is right? Experiments in thinking about the process of infant feeding generate at least two cultural models—one of breastfeeding and one of bottle feeding (Holland and Quinn 1987). Cultural models frame experience, have directive force, occur at different levels of abstraction, and include general purpose, folk, and expert models (Holland and Quinn 1987). Interpretations of infant feeding may be guided by models of breastfeeding or models of bottle feeding. Let us call these hypothetical models general purpose models of breastfeeding and bottle feeding. Note that these general purpose models may have wide applicability and may bear little relation to expert models of each.

Although these models are culturally constructed, simplified schemata may underlie both models. It is likely that cross-culturally there are significant similarities between both breastfeeding and bottle feeding models. Similarities in breastfeeding models exist because cultural models build on the same biological processes of milk production and ejection and the resulting biosocial link between mother and infant. This biosocial link rapidly becomes embedded in culturally and historically defined social relations, producing a number of different breastfeeding styles (see Van Esterik and Elliott 1986; Van Esterik 1985b).

Artificial feeding, on the other hand, may be interpreted by reference to a breastfeeding model or to a separately constructed bottle feeding model that is unrelated to any biological processes. In this case, promotion and advertising play an important role in shaping the similarities between cultural models of bottle feeding cross-culturally.

These cultural models organize knowledge and frame the experience of infant feeding in radically different ways. The cognitive orientations developed here relate closely to those contrasts defined by Berger (1973) for modernity, and Bloom (1981) on the power of breastfeeding. Yet both argue that these cognitive orientations carry over into other domains of life. This is characteristic of general purpose models that apply to multiple domains of life. Table 6.1 contrasts these orientations.

Breastfeeding Model. The breastfeeding model develops from the model of renewable resources. As a renewable resource, breastfeeding operates on the satiation principle stressing non-measurable criteria like satisfaction. In this model, as demand increases, supply increases. Time orientation is to cyclical, recurrent rhythms, reinforcing the continuity between the reproductive phases of pregnancy, birth, lactation, and weaning. Breastfeeding is an individualized process; breastmilk is a living, changing product adapted to the age of the child and the microenvironment of the mother. The primary social links formed are highly personalized links between mother and infant, or more rarely between another female adult and an infant. Most significant, in the breastfeeding model the infant is active and in control of the process. It is thus a newborn's first experience of empowerment.

Bottle Feeding Model. The bottle feeding model develops from the use of nonrenewable resources. Bottle feeding operates on the scarcity principle, reinforcing the idea of limited good and the fact that resources can be used up. As demand increases, supply decreases, resulting in a stress on quantity and measurement. Time, too, must be measured and divided into components, sequences, and schedules. Infant formula, the most appropriate breastmilk substitute, is a standardized prod-

TABLE 6.1
Cultural models of infant feeding

Breastfeeding Model	*Bottle Feeding/Infant Formula Model*
Renewable resource	Nonrenewable resource
Living product	Inert substance
Satiation principle (as demand increases, the supply increases)	Scarcity principle (limited good, as demand increases, supply decreases)
Nonmeasurable (stress on satisfaction)	Measurable (stress on quantity)
Orientation to time: reinforcement of continuity between reproductive phases (pregnancy, birth lactation, weaning)	Orientation to time: divisible into components and measurable sequences
Cyclical recurrent rhythms	Scheduling
Individualized process (adapted to age of child, viruses of mother, etc.)	Standardized product (formula for a constantly improving product)
Personalized primary links between mother and infant (or rarely other adult female)	Generalized primary links with any male or female, adult or child
Infant is active and in control	Infant is passive and controlled by others
Empowerment	Dependency (consumer from birth)

uct, constantly being improved in an effort to replicate human milk. The process of bottle feeding encourages the formation of generalized social links, as bottle feeding can be accomplished by males or females, adults or children. During bottle feeding, the infant is passive and controlled by others, providing the newborn's first experience of dependency and creating a consumer from birth.

Note that in Table 6.1 the second model is labeled bottle feeding/infant formula model. Epidemiological survey data must distinguish carefully between bottle feeding as a mode of feeding and infant formula as only one of many possible products that could be fed by bottle or cup and spoon. However, a cultural model can reflect the more common-sense observation that infant formula and feeding bottles are clearly linked in people's minds and are reinforced by visual and printed copy in advertisements. It is likely that this second model did not gain cognitive saliency until proprietary formulas were popular in North America around the turn of the century.

In different societies throughout history, the breastfeeding model was probably overgeneralized to cover all modes of infant feeding. Bottle feeding as a new process would probably have been understood by reference to the known process of lactation. By analogy, the bottle becomes a portable breast. When the breastfeeding model is conceptually extended to cover bottle feeding, a number of problems result from assuming that a breastfed baby is "like" a bottle fed baby (see Chapter Five).

When bottle feeding dominated, as in many North American contexts in the forties and fifties, lactation was poorly understood and interpreted by reference to the dominant bottle feeding model. The "bottled breast" had to be emptied out, cleaned off, and scheduled, to the detriment of breastfeeding. The bottle feeding model is constantly reinforced when medical practitioners assume that infant formula is equivalent to, or even better than human milk. The idea that bottle feeding and breastfeeding are equivalent is a prime example of what Bateson would call an error in thinking.

Hypothetically it should be possible for the two models to

coexist in one community or even in the mind of an individual woman. However, the contradictions arising from the two models may simply increase mothers' concerns about infant feeding in general. These two models coexist in Bogotà where bottle feeding is common. Yet, the breastfeeding model of infant feeding is influential as mothers constantly try to individualize their infants' bottle feeding, adjusting herbs, brown sugar, and milk to achieve the correct balance to suit the age, individual temperament, and health of their children.

Neither the breastfeeding nor bottle feeding model is static. Recently, breastfeeding promotion campaigns have stressed the protective power of breastmilk. But this concept may emerge not from indigenous ideas about the power of breastmilk as a product (including magical beliefs that breastmilk cures eye diseases), but from the idea that infant formula offers magical protection for infants. Mothers like Rosa's neighbor, who breastfed her child only to have her die, are unlikely to believe in the protective power of breastmilk, no matter how much effort and money is expended on breastfeeding promotion.

Future Trajectories

Policies are courses of action adopted as advantageous or expedient for the conduct of public affairs. Although infant feeding policy is not the responsibility of activists, during the course of the controversy, certain policy directions for infant feeding were clarified, if not simplied. Dilemmas emerged during the debates concerning definitions of maternal depletion, small but healthy infants, and infants that "have to be fed" infant formula. Policy decisions require imagining distant goals and creating strategies for reaching them. The courses of action adopted as the most expedient means to influence decision-making guide the conduct of key sectors such as health, population, or industry. There are few institutions in the world system that can address global infant feeding policy. It is only at the world-system level that infant feeding patterns can be seen to be embedded in their broadest contexts. But there are many institutions at the national level that can set policies for improving infant feeding. The two hypothetical trajectories developed here project the future impact of possible changes in infant feeding patterns at the national level. When policy-makers choose the most valued scenario for their countries, then consistent strategies for reaching that goal can be developed.

First, let us consider a scenario where (1) the breastfeeding model is the dominant or exclusive cognitive model used by both laymen and experts to interpret infant feeding, and (2) where all systems must accommodate a large breastfeeding population (compared with current rates of initiation, duration, and frequency). The second scenario reverses these conditions: (1) the bottle feeding model dominates and is the dominant or exclusive cognitive model used by both laymen and experts to interpret infant feeding, and (2) all systems must accommodate a large bottle feeding population (compared with current rates of initiation, duration, and frequency). The following scenarios should help us identify forces potentially supportive of breastfeeding and bottle feeding.

SCENARIO 1: Breastfeeding Trajectory
Sustainable Environments

1. Utilization of renewable resources, therefore no strain on ecosystem
2. No production of solid wastes
3. Lessened demand for fuel supplies

4. Pressure for clean water supply to improve women's health status
5. Links between living conditions and infant morbidity and mortality are direct and can easily be made obvious to mothers
6. Greater pressure to reduce dangers of radiation in environment
7. Greater pressure to reduce environmental pollutants

SCENARIO 2: Bottle Feeding Trajectory
Sustainable Environments

1. Utilization of nonrenewable resources to produce and prepare infant formula, therefore strain on ecosystem
2. Production of solid wastes
3. Increased demand for fuel supplies
4. Pressures for clean water supply to prepare adequate breastmilk substitutes
5. Links between living conditions and infant morbidity and mortality are less direct and harder to demonstrate to mothers
6. Less pressure to reduce dangers of radiation in environment
7. Less pressure to reduce environmental pollutants

SCENARIO 1: Breastfeeding Trajectory
Empowerment of Women

1. Mothers and infants control infant feeding
2. Death/illness of mother puts infant in jeopardy, therefore increased pressure to reduce maternal morbidity and mortality
3. Need for postpartum period of recovery, rest after childbirth, and support from other women

4. Need for increase in quality and quantity of food for new mothers (often through special diets)
5. Delay in return to full-time work pattern
6. Work pattern changes, e.g., constrained by periodicity
7. More pressure for maternity leaves, creches, and lactation breaks for women employed outside the home
8. Necessity to reduce emotional and physical stress on women
9. Cigarette smoking potentially detrimental to breastfeeding, therefore pressure on women to reduce cigarette smoking
10. Increase in child spacing and increased pressure for safe contraception that does not affect lactation

SCENARIO 2: Bottle Feeding Trajectory
Empowerment of Women

1. Adults or children control infant feeding
2. Death/illness of mother does not put infant in jeopardy, therefore less pressure to reduce maternal morbidity and mortality
3. No postpartum period of recovery and rest necessary; no support from other women necessary
4. No special diets or increase in food supply needed for new mothers
5. Immediate return to full-time work possible
6. Work pattern not constrained by periodicity
7. Less pressure for maternity leaves and creches for women employed outside the home
8. No pressure or necessity to reduce emotional and physical stress on women
9. Cigarette smoking irrelevant to bottle feeding, therefore no pressure on women to reduce smoking
10. Decrease in child spacing and increased need for contra-

ceptives (no concerns about contraception affecting infants)

SCENARIO 1: Breastfeeding Trajectory
Medicalization

1. Breastfeeding "mishaps" rare because of greater understanding of and support for breastfeeding (stained clothes are a common example of a breastfeeding "mishap"); no medical consequences for an individual woman who "fails" at breastfeeding (personal disappointment with no wider consequences)
2. Decreased dependence on doctors
3. Increased dependence on women's support groups (like La Leche League or local variants) and lactation advisers (paraprofessionals)
4. Changing morbidity patterns include possible decrease in food allergies, dental caries, kidney diseases, infantile obesity, and SIDS
5. Decreased importance of pharmaceutical companies in the health system
6. Hospital routines geared to breastfeeding, e.g., more facilities for early contact between mothers and infants; more facilities for rooming-in; more facilities for drug-free nonintrusive childbirth; more facilities for feeding on demand

SCENARIO 2: Bottle Feeding Trajectory
Medicalization

1. Infant formula "mishaps" common from industrial accidents; serious medical consequences for infant and potential wider community consequences if defect is not discovered quickly, e.g., bacterial contamination; defective formula (too much salt, iron, iodine, fluoride, or

lead; or not enough zinc, selenium, chloride, biotin, cysteine, or taurine)
2. Increased dependence on doctors to advise on suitable infant formula and to cure problems infants develop as a consequence of consuming infant formula
3. Decreased importance of women's support groups and other paraprofessionals such as lactation advisers
4. Changing morbidity patterns include possible increase in food allergies, dental caries, kidney diseases, infantile obesity, and SIDS
5. Closer relations between medical systems and pharmaceutical and food companies producing infant formula
6. Hospital routines geared to bottle feeding, e.g., fewer pressures for early contact, rooming-in, drug-free birth, or demand feeding

SCENARIO 1: Breastfeeding Trajectory
Commoditization of Food

1. Less dependency on delocalized food resources
2. Reduction of competitive marketing and advertising environment
3. Emphasis on food as a human right

SCENARIO 2: Bottle Feeding Trajectory
Commoditization of Food

1. Greater dependency on delocalized food resources
2. Dependence on advertising and marketing to alter market shares of competing infant formula companies
3. Emphasis on food as commodity

The most important observations following from the construction of these two trajectories are the immense differences in the scale of the potential problems associated with increased breastfeeding or bottle feeding, and the forces potentially supportive of each. There are no negative consequences associated with the breastfeeding trajectory and many negative consequences and unknown risks related to the bottle feeding trajectory. Minchin refers to artificial feeding as the largest uncontrolled in vivo experiment in human history (1985:316). The key point is that we know very little about the long-term intergenerational effects of artificial feeding—on food allergies or autoimmune diseases, for example. The forces potentially supportive of the breastfeeding trajectory include those advocacy groups concerned with reducing environmental pollution, dependency on pharmaceutical products, and risks of nuclear contamination. The forces potentially supportive of the bottle feeding/infant formula trajectory include food and drug companies and employers who exploit women's labor.

Infant Feeding and Sustainable Development

Among the many competing views of development, Another Development stands out as a conceptual model capable of explaining the implications of different infant feeding patterns. Another Development is "people-centred, geared to the satisfaction of human needs—both material and in the broadest sense, political; it is self-reliant, endogenous, ecologically sound and based on democratic, political, social, and economic structural transformations" (Hammarskjöld 1975)

Another Development begins with the analysis of concrete situations like infant feeding. Breastfeeding is the epitome of an activity that is "people-centred" rather than technology based; it is geared solely to the satisfaction of the needs of both mother and infant; the majority of the population would improve both their nutritional and health status through increased breastfeeding, while only an elite minority can benefit from bottle feeding. Increased breastfeeding fulfills certain political objectives by reducing dependency on multinational corporations and decreasing their influence in the health sector. Breastfeeding strengthens self-reliance by reducing dependence on external institutions and products, and the product is certainly produced locally. It is ecologically sound. Unlike infant formula and bottle feeding, which utilize nonrenewable resources, breastfeeding only requires investing in the health of the mother. Although breastfeeding is essentially a conservative mammalian function, it requires radical social structural transformations to succeed. These include changes in the division of labor, more equitable distribution of income and resources, and higher priorities on maternal and child welfare. Improved maternal health, then, is a prerequisite for policies encouraging breastfeeding. From the perspective of Another Development, it is very shortsighted to argue that policies encouraging breastfeeding are infant centered and policies encouraging bottle feeding are mother centered.

Sustainable development, like Another Development, proposes a new approach to development—one that focuses attention on the environmental resource base. Sustainable development is "a process of change in which the exploitation of resources, the direction of investments, the orientation of technological development, and institutional change are made consistent with future as well as present needs" (World Commission on Environment and Development 1987:9). This approach emphasizes the need to reconcile current with future potential to meet human needs for both developing and developed countries. In both the short and long run, policies encouraging breastfeeding must benefit both mothers and infants and ultimately contribute to sustainable development.

It is tempting to say that the choice is clear and simple—that the breastfeeding trajectory is the desired future scenario and that all policy initiatives should emphasize the need for consistent efforts in that direction, with the objective of having more women initiate breastfeeding and breastfeed for longer duration. In fact, these may be short-term objectives and—as the lives of Rosa, Grace, Sunoto, and Amporn illustrate—not all that easily accomplished. Such objectives represent incomplete accounting and set the stage for blaming mothers for not breastfeeding successfully. By framing the breast-bottle controversy around the issues of poverty environments, empowerment of women, medicalization of infant feeding, and the commoditization of food, attention is shifted away from the infant feeding decisions of individual mothers and on to the conditions affecting their decisions and lives.

The trajectory goal becomes not to have every woman breastfeed her infant, but to create conditions in individuals, households, communities, and nations so that every women could. The first step is to create conditions that make breastfeeding possible, successful, and valued in a given society.

One obstacle to setting this as a policy objective is that the implications arising from this position include broad social, economic, and political transformations far removed from usual infant feeding policy decisions. The United States recognized these broad implications arising from the adoption of the WHO/UNICEF Code and refused to support it because it threatened the operation of multinational corporations, particularly American multinationals. Repercussions are even more likely to occur in third world contexts where citizen action groups may be viewed as a real threat to national security. Advocacy groups are not always prepared to take on these larger agendas, and certainly anthropologists seldom are. Harries-Jones argues that "advocacy anthropology in Third World contexts all too easily becomes tied to advocacy for total social and political transformation, and anthropologists find it difficult to extract themselves from arguments for total transformation" (1985:233). It is enough to give up one brand of coffee or donate to an activist group without advocating total social transformation!

ADVOCACY AND RESEARCH DISCOURSES

> The infant formula controversy has meant different things to different people. To many health professionals and public health administrators, it was a crusade for improvement in infant and young child health. To some activists, it was a campaign against the power and influence of multinational business corporations. To church leaders and members, the conflict was an opportunity to raise moral consciousness about the problems of world hunger. To leaders in business and government, at the national and international levels, it has sometimes seemed a holy war against the infant formula industry, if not a challenge to free enterprise and capitalism itself. To the optimists, the emergence of the World Health Organization Code of Marketing for Breastmilk Substitutes has been an opportunity for industry and government to collaborate on the improvement of the human condition. To the pessimists, including a few in the Reagan Administration, the Code has seemed a dangerous and precedent-setting foray into international regulation. Few issues have given more credence to the proposition that political meaning, like art, is to be found in the eye of the beholder. (Post 1985:113)

These different perspectives identified by Post are grounded in different values and assumptions, although they are all ultimately connected with each other. Interpreting the infant formula controversy requires unraveling the relations and contradictions between these different views. Like other human rights and justice issues, the problem underlying the breast-bottle controversy remains a divergent one. Other consumer rights groups have been formed around related issues such as the promotion of pharmaceutical products (Health Action International), pollution (Pollution Probe), and pesticides (Pesticide Action Group), all organized out of the International Organization of Consumer Unions, the home of IBFAN. The focus of each group may be different, but the themes of manipulation and waste and the strategies to combat the greed of multinational corporations are familiar to the activists who worked on the infant formula controversy. Advocacy groups appear to treat "causes" as convergent problems in order to take action. Thus, they tend to oversimplify complexities. Advocacy action may not always be linked to organized social movements. Rosenberg writes that

> such groups, by their very existence, provide lived alternatives to the alienating and oppressive conditions around them. Because they are usually composed of society's less powerful people, they are rarely taken seriously by those with power. Such grass-roots groups are like social guerrillas who deal in localized hit and run operations not full-fledged battles. But herein may lie their advantage. They are harder for the structure of rule to locate, co-opt, or eradicate. They may be suppressed in one place but reform and reappear in another. (1986:100)

In the practice of advocacy, the complexities are revealed. For some people this requires pulling out of immediate practical action to grapple with these emergent theoretical issues. For others, these complexities confuse and frustrate, and lead to early "burn-out," which is inevitable considering the intensity of commitment of many activists. Fortunately, some retain the single-mindedness to pursue even limited objectives—rephrasing and translating part of the WHO/UNICEF Code, exploring funding histories of research groups, demanding labeling changes on cans of infant formula sold in one country.

Advocacy discourse reduces problems to simple convergent problems in order to take action; taking action reveals the complexity of the embedded divergent problems. Ironically, research discourse encourages the reverse. Issues begin as complex divergent questions phrased in a complex academic communicative code. Through the course of data collection and analysis, the complexities are often reduced to simple convergent questions, as contexts are reduced to background variables and results further reduced statistically. Rather than directing social action, research often begets more data collection, more details, a finer analysis—more research.

Harries-Jones (1985) argues that advocacy is not merely the application of knowledge acquired through research, as traditional applied anthropology assumes, but rather the interpretation of practical knowledge-in-use from which theoretical insights can be drawn. The advocacy discourse was critically important to the recent policy initiatives on infant feeding, such as the WHO/UNICEF Code. Knowledge about the advantages of breastfeeding and the consequences of bottle feeding was available long before the publicity of the seventies. Advocacy action was needed rather than more research or another task force. Knowledge is not the problem; the problem is an "unwillingness to use what is already known for the benefit of women or social justice. There is unwillingness to use what is known about power inequalities for the redistribution of power" (Maguire 1984:50).

Anthropologists have an important contribution to make to advocacy discourse, for they are often the possessors of knowledge that can be used for change or stasis. Their methods are most likely to reveal linkages between macrostructures operating in the world system and the minutiae of everyday life. But to maintain the will and commitment to put this knowledge to use, we need the idealistic rhetoric of the committed advocate as a reminder to ask significant questions. Mies asks, "what would a society be like in which women, nature and colonies were not exploited in the name of the accumulation of ever more wealth and money" (1986:205)? If we cannot imagine the alternative, then we cannot contribute to its construction.

Bibliography

Adelman, C. 1983. "Infant Formula, Science and Politics." *Policy Review* 23: 107–126.

American Public Health Association. 1986. *Government Legislation and Policies to Support Breastfeeding, Improve Maternal and Infant Nutrition, and Implement a Code of Marketing of Breastmilk Substitutes.* Report No 4, Washington, D.C.

Anderson, M. 1985. "Technology Implications for Women." In *Gender Roles in Development Projects: A Case Book,* edited by C. Overholt, M. Anderson, K. Cloud, and J. Austin. West Hartford, Conn.: Kumarian Press.

Apple, R. 1980. "To be Used Only Under the Direction of a Physician: Commercial Infant Feeding and Medical Practice, 1870–1940." *Journal of the History of Medicine* 54: 402–417.

Arneil, G. 1983. "Role of Food Industry in Promoting Human Nutrition: The Pediatrician's Point of View." *Proceedings of the Asian Conference of Nutrition,* Bangkok, Thailand.

Baer, H., M. Singer and J. H. Johnson. 1986. "Toward a

Critical Medical Anthroplogy." *Social Science and Medicine* 23(2): 95–98.

Barnett, H. G. 1953. *Innovation: The Basis of Cultural Change.* New York: McGraw-Hill.

Bateson, G. 1972. *Steps to an Ecology of Mind.* New York: Ballantine Books.

Baudrillard, J. 1981. *For a Critique of the Political Economy of the Sign.* St. Louis: Telos Press.

Benarde, M. 1973. *Our Precarious Habitat.* New York: W. W. Norton and Company Inc.

Benería, L., and G. Sen. 1982. "Class and Gender Inequalities and Women's Role in Economic Development: Theoretical and Practical Implications." *Feminist Studies* 8(1): 157–176.

Berg, A. 1973. *The Nutrition Factor.* Washington, D.C.: Brookings Institution.

Berger, P., B. Berger, and H. Kellner. 1984. *The Homeless Mind.* New York: Vintage Books.

Biddulph, J. 1980. "Impact of Legislation Restricting the Availability of Feeding Bottles in Papua new Guinea." *Nutrition and Development* 3(2): 4–6.

Blackman, L. 1981. "Dancing in the Dark. Helping and Not So Helping Hands." *Birth and the Family Journal* 8(4): 280–286.

Bloom, B. S. 1979. "Stretching Ideology to the Utmost. Marxism and Medical Technology." *American Journal of Public Health* 69(12): 1269–1279.

Bloom, M. 1981. "The Romance and Power of Breastfeeding." *Birth and the Family Journal* 8(4): 259–269.

Borgoltz, P. 1979. "Economic and Business Aspects of Infant Formula Promotion: Implications for Nutrition Policy in Developing Countries." Report to UNICEF and WHO.

Boulding, E., J. Passmore, and R. Gassler. 1976. *Handbook of International Data on Women.* New York: John Wiley and Sons.

Bourdieu, P. 1984. *Distinction: A Social Critique of the Judge-*

ment of Taste. Translated by R. Nice. Cambridge, Mass.: Harvard University Press.

Bovornsiri, V. 1982. "Role, Status, and Problems of Women in Education Development: Thailand." In *Women in Development: Implications for Population Dynamics in Thailand*. edited by S. Prasith-rathsint and S. Piampiti. Bangkok: National Institute for Development Administration.

Brack, D. C. 1979. "Why Women Breast-Feed." Ph.D. diss. City University of New York.

Browner, C., and E. Lewin. 1982. "Female Altruism Reconsidered: The Virgin Mary as Economic Woman." *American Ethnologist* 9(1): 61–75.

Campbell, C. 1984. "Nestle and Breast vs Bottle Feeding: Mainstream and Marxist Perspectives." *International Journal of Health Services* 14(4): 547–567.

Cappon, D. 1971. *Technology and Perception*. Springfield, Ill.: Charles C. Thomas.

Cassidy, C. 1987. "World View, Conflict and Toddler Malnutrition: Change Agent Dilemmas." In *Child Survival*, edited by N. Scheper-Hughes. Dordrecht: D. Reidel.

Chambers, R. 1977 *Rural Development. Putting the Last First*. London: Longman.

Chetley, A. 1986. *The Politics of Baby Food*. London: Frances Pinter.

Chrisman, N. J., and T. W. Maretzki. 1982. *Clinically Applied Anthropology*. Dordrecht: D. Reidel.

Clarkson, F. 1983. "Formula for Funding." *Fairfield County Advocate*. May 4.

Collar, M. 1978. "The Pablum Connection." *Toronto Star Sunday Magazine*. Dec. 17.

Conrad, P., and J. Schneider. 1980. *Deviance and Medicalization: From Badness to Sickness*. St. Louis: C. V. Mosby Co.

———. 1986. "Professionalization, Monopoly, and the Structure of Medical Practice." In *Sociology of Health and Illness*, edited by P. Conrad and R. Kern. New York: St. Martin's Press.

Cosminski, S. 1985. "Infant Feeding Practices in Rural Kenya." In *Breastfeeding, Child Health, and Child Spacing,* edited by V. Hull and M. Simpson. London: Croom Helm.

Craddock, V. M. 1981. "Environmental Nitrosamines and Cancer." *Nature* 294: 694–695.

Csikszentmihalyi, M., and E. Rochberg-Halton. 1981. *The Meaning of Things.* Cambridge: Cambridge University Press.

Donaldson, P. 1981. "Foreign Intervention in Medical Education: A Case Study of the Rockefeller Foundation's Involvement in a Thai Medical School." *International Journal of Health Services* 6(2): 251–269.

Douglas, M., and B. Asherwood. 1979. *The World of Goods.* New York: Basic Books.

Drake, T. G. 1948. "American Infant Feeding Bottles 1841–1946." *Journal of the History of Medicine* 3(Autumn): 507–524.

DuBois, Cora. 1941. "Attitudes Toward Food and Hunger in Alor." In *Language, Culture, and Personality,* edited by L. Spier, A. Hallowell, and S. Newman. Menasha, Wis.: Sapir Memorial Publication Fund.

Duley, E. 1986. *The Cross Cultural Study of Women.* New York: Feminist Press.

Ehrenreich, J., ed. 1978. *The Cultural Crisis of Modern Medicine.* New York and London: Monthly Review Press.

Ehrenreich, B., and D. English. 1979. *For Her Own Good.* Garden City, N.Y.: Anchor Books.

Eisenberg, L., and A. Kleinman. 1981. "Clinical Social Science." In *The Relevance of Social Science for Medicine,* edited by L. Eisenberg and A. Kleinman. Dordrecht: D. Reidel.

Eisenstein, H. 1983. *Contemporary Feminist Thought:* Boston: G. K. Hall.

Evans, P. 1967. "Fashions in Infant Feeding." *A Symposium on the Child,* edited by J. A. Askin, R. E. Cooke, and J. A. Haller, Jr. Baltimore: The Johns Hopkins University Press.

Evans, S. 1980. "Breastfeeding." *Spare Rib* (December): 49–52.

Everett, R. ed. 1962. *Diffusion of Innovations.* New York: Glencoe Free Press.

Ewen, S. 1976. *Captains of Consciousness: Advertising and the Social Roots of Consumer Culture.* New York: McGraw-Hill.

Fawcett, J., S. Khoo, and P. Smith. 1984. *Women in the Cities of Asia.* Boulder, Col.: Westview Press.

Feldman, M. S., and J. G. March. 1981. "Information in Organizations as Signal and Symbol." *Administrative Science Quarterly* 26: 171–186.

Fildes, V. 1986. *Breasts, Bottles and Babies.* Edinburgh: Edinburgh University Press.

Fisher, B. 1984. "Guilt and Shame in the Women's Movement: The Radical Ideal of Action and its Meaning for Feminist Intellectuals." *Feminist Studies* 10(2): 185–212.

Ford, C. 1980. *Charlotte Ford's Book of Modern Manners.* New York: Simon and Schuster.

Foucault, M. 1980. *Power/Knowledge; Selected Interviews and Other Writings, 1972–1977,* translated by C. Gordon. New York: Pantheon.

Freedman, M. 1955. *A Report on Some Aspects of Food, Health, and Society in Indonesia.* Geneva: World Health Organization.

Freidson, E. 1970. *Professional Dominance. The Structure of Medical Care.* New York: Atherton Press.

Furedi, F. 1973. "The African Crowd in Nairobi: Popular Movements and Elite Politics." *Journal of African History* 14: 275–290.

Gardner, B. B., and S. J. Levy. 1955. "The Product and the Brand." *Harvard Business Review* 33 (March–April): 33–39.

Gaskin, I. M. 1987. *Babies, Breastfeeding, and Bonding.* South Hadley, Mass.: Bergin and Garvey Publishers.

Geertz, C. 1983. "Blurred Genres: The Refiguration of Social Thought." In *Local Knowledge: Further Essays in Interpretive Anthropology*, by Clifford Geertz. New York: Basic Books.

George, S. 1977. *How the Other Half Dies*. Montclair, N.J.: Allanheld, Osmun and Co.

Gerlach, L. P. 1980. "The Flea and the Elephant: Infant Formula Controversy." *Transaction* 17(6): 51–57.

Goody, J. 1982. *Cooking, Cuisine and Class*. Cambridge: Cambridge University Press.

Gordon, L. 1978. "The Politics of Birth Control 1920–1940. The Impact of Professionals." In *The Cultural Crisis of Modern Medicine*, edited by J. Ehrenreich. New York: Monthly Review Press.

Gottdiener, M. 1985. "Hegemony and Mass Culture: A Semiotic Approach." *American Journal of Sociology* 80(5): 978–1001.

Greiner, T. 1982. "Infant Feeding Policy Options for Governments." Report for the USAID Funded Infant Feeding Consortium. New York: Population Council.

Greiner, T., P. Van Esterik, and M. Latham. 1981. "The Insufficient Milk Syndrome: An Alternative Explanation." *Medical Anthropology* 5(2): 233–247.

Gussler, J., and L. Briesemeister. 1980. "The Insufficient Milk Syndrome: A Biocultural Explanation." *Medical Anthropology* 4(2): 145–174.

Haller, T. 1983. *Danger: Marketing Researcher at Work*. Westport, Conn.: Quorum Books.

Hallman, D. 1985. "Reflections on the Nestle Boycott." *Food and Development. CUSO Journal* (July): 59–61.

Hammarskjöld, Dag. 1975. *What Now: Another Development*. Dag Hammarskjöld Centre Report. Uppsala, Sweden.

Hanks, L., and J. Hanks. 1963. "Thailand: Equality Between the Sexes." In *Women in the New Asia*, edited by B. Ward. Paris: UNESCO.

Hardyment, C. 1983. *Dream Babies*. London: Jonathan Cape.

Harevern, T. 1982. *Family Time and Industrial Time.* Cambridge: Cambridge University Press.

Harries-Jones, P. 1985. "From Cultural Translator to Advocate: Changing Circles of Interpretation." In *Advocacy and Anthropology,* edited by R. Paine. St. John's, Newfoundland: Institute of Social and Economic Research.

Hart, H., M. Bax, and S. Jenkins. 1980. "Community Influences on Breastfeeding." *Child Care, Health, and Development* 6: 175–187.

Haschke, F., B. Pietschnig, V. Karg, H. Vanura, and E. Schuster. 1987. "Letter to the Editor." *New England Journal of Medicine* 316: 409–410.

Helsing, E. 1979. "Women's Liberation and Breastfeeding." In *Lactation, Fertility and the Working Woman,* edited by D. B. Jelliffe. London: International Planned Parenthood Federation.

Henderson, J. W. 1986. "The New International Division of Labour and American Semiconductor Production in Southeast Asia." In *Multinational Corporations and the Third World,* edited by C. J. Dixon, D. Drakakis-Smith, and H. D. Watts. Boulder, Col.: Westview Press.

Hesch, J. W. 1948. *The Hygiene Study Ward Centre at Batavia (1937–1941).* Scholae Medicinae Tropicae, 19, Leiden.

Higginbotham, H. 1984. *Third World Challenge to Psychiatry.* East-West Center: University of Hawaii Press.

Hofvander, Y. 1979. "Scandanavian Case Study." In *Lactation, Fertility and the Working Women,* edited by D. B. Jelliffe. London: International Planned Parenthood Federation.

Holland, D., and N. Quinn. 1987. *Cultural Models in Language and Thought.* Cambridge: Cambridge University Press.

Human Lactation Center. 1977. "Mothers in Poverty." *Lactation Review* 2(3): 1–19.

Illich, I. 1976. *Medical Nemesis.* New York: Pantheon Books.

Jaggar, A. 1983. *Feminist Politics and Human Nature.* Totowa, N.J.: Rowman and Allanheld.

Jayasuriya, D., A. Griffiths, and R. Rigoni. 1984. *Judgement*

Reserved. Breast-feeding, Bottle-feeding, and the International Code. Sri Lanka: Nedimala Dehivala.

Jelliffe, D. B., and E.F.P. Jelliffe. 1978. *Human Milk in the Modern World*. Oxford: Oxford University Press.

Joseph, S. 1981. "The Infant Formula Controversy: An International Health Policy Paradigm." *Annals of Internal Medicine* 95(3): 383–384.

Kaplinsky, R. 1981. "Inappropriate Products and Techniques in Underdeveloped Countries: The Case of Breakfast Foods in Kenya." In *Methods for Development Planning*. Paris: UNESCO Press.

Kettel, B. 1986. "Women in Kenya at the End of the U.N. Decade." *Canadian Woman Studies Journal* 7: 38–41.

King, C. W. 1964. "Fashion Adoption: A Rebuttal to the Trickle Down Theory." In *Toward Scientific Marketing*, edited by S. A. Greysen. Chicago: American Marketing Association.

Kleinman, A. 1980. *Patients and Healers in the Context of Culture*. Berkeley: University of California Press.

Kleinman, A., L. Eisenberg, and B. Good. 1978. "Culture, Illness and Care. Clinical Lessons from Anthropological and Cross Cultural Research." *Annals of Internal Medicine* 88: 251–258.

Knodel, J. 1982. "Breastfeeding in Thailand; Data from the 1981 Contraceptive Prevalence Survey." *Studies in Family Planning* 13(11): 307–315.

La Leche League. 1976. *The Womanly Art of Breastfeeding*. Franklin Park, Ill.

Lall, L., and S. Bibile. 1981. "The Political Economy of Controlling Transnationals in the Pharmaceutical Industry in Sri Lanka." In *Imperialism, Health and Medicine*, edited by V. Narvarro. New York: Baywood Publishers.

Landon, E. 1974. "Self Concept, Ideal Self Concept and Consumer Purchase Intentions." *Journal of Consumer Research* 1: 44–51.

Langdon, S. 1975. "Multinational Corporations, Taste Transfer, and Underdevelopment: A Case Study from Kenya." *Review of African Political Economy* 2: 12–35.

Lappé, F. M., and J. Collins. 1977. *Food First*. Boston: Houghton Mifflin.

Latham, M. C. 1964. "Nutritional Problems of Tanganyika." In: *Proceedings of Sixth International Congress of Nutrition, Edinburgh, 9th to 15th August 1963*. Edinburgh: E. and S. Livingstone.

———. 1965. *Human Nutrition in Tropical Africa*. Rome: Food and Agriculture Organization of U.N.

———. 1975. "Introduction." In *The Promotion of Bottle Feeding by Multi National Corporations: How Advertising and the Health Professions have Contributed,* T. Greiner. Cornell Monograph Series in International Nutrition, No. 2. Ithaca, N.Y.

———. 1978. "Nutrition and Culture." In *Nutrition and National Policy,* edited by B. Winikoff. Cambridge: MIT Press.

———. 1988. "Maternal and Infant Nutrition—An International Perspective." In *The Pacific Conference. Nutrition Challenges in a Changing World,* edited by M. Bruss. Honolulu: Hawaii Nutrition Council and Society for Nutrition Education.

Latham, M. C., T. C. Elliott, B. Winikoff, J. Kekovole, and P. Van Esterik. 1986. "Infant Feeding in Urban Kenya: A Pattern of Early Triple Nipple Feeding." *Journal of Tropical Pediatrics* 32: 276–280.

Lazer, W. 1964. "Life Style Concepts and Marketing." In *Toward Scientific Marketing,* edited by S. A. Greysen. Chicago: A. Mark Associates.

Lazer, W., and E. Kelley. 1973. *Social Marketing*. Homewood, Ill.: Richard D. Ariven Inc.

Leiss, W., S. Kline, and S. Jhally. 1986. *Social Communication in Advertising*. Toronto: Methuen Press.

Lexchin, J. 1984. *The Real Pushers*. Vancouver: New Star Books.

Lock, M. 1986. "Plea for Acceptance: School Refusal Syndrome in Japan." *Social Science and Medicine* 2: 99–112.

Maguire, P. 1984. *Women in Development: An Alternative Analysis*. Center for International Education, University of Massachusetts.

Manderson, L. 1982. "Bottle Feeding and Ideology in Colonial Malaya: The Production of Change." *International Journal of Health Services* 12(4): 597–616.

———. 1983. "Introduction." In *Women's Work and Women's Roles: Economics and Everyday Life in Indonesia, Malaysia, and Singapore,* edited by L. Manderson. Development Studies Centre, Monograph No. 33. Canberra: Australian National University.

Martin, E. 1987. *The Woman in the Body*. Boston: Beacon Press.

Mascia-Lees, F. 1984. *Towards a Model of Women's Status*. New York: Peter Lang.

Mattelart, A. 1983. *Transnationals and the Third World*. South Hadley, Mass.: Bergin and Garvey Publishers.

McCaffery, M. 1984. "Breastfeeding: Religious Experience or Hard Work." *Canadian Family Physician* 30: 1441–1442.

McCracken, G. 1986. "Culture and Consumption: A Theoretical Account of the Structure and Movement of the Cultural Meaning of Consumer Goods." *Journal of Consumer Research* 13: 71–84.

McGee, T. 1975. *Food Dependency in the Pacific: A Preliminary Statement*. Research School of Pacific Research Studies (2). Australian National University.

McKeown, T. 1979. *The Role of Medicine: Dream, Mirage or Nemesis*. Princeton: Princeton University Press.

McMichael, J. K., ed. 1976. *Health and the Third World*. Nottingham: Spokesman Books.

Meador, C. 1965. "The Art and Science of Non-Disease." *New England Journal of Medicine* 277: 92–95.

Meesook, A. 1978. "Cultures in Collision. An Experience of Thailand." In *Culture in Encounter,* ASEAN Cultural Week, Tubingen, Germany.

Mies, M. 1986. *Patriarchy and Accumulation on a World Scale.* London: Zed Press.

Minchin, M. 1985. *Breastfeeding Matters.* Sydney, Australia: George Allen and Unwin.

Morgan, M., M. Calman, and N. Manning. 1985. *Sociological Approaches to Health and Medicine.* London: Croom Helm.

Morgan, R. 1984. *Sisterhood is Global.* Garden City, N.Y.: Anchor Press.

Muecke, M. 1976. "Health Care Systems as Socializing Agents: Childbearing the North Thai and Western Ways." *Social Science and Medicine* 10: 377–383.

Mulder, N. 1978. *Everyday Life in Thailand.* Bangkok: D. K. Press.

Muller, M. *The Baby Killer.* London: War on Want.

Navarro, V. 1976. *Medicine Under Capitalism.* London: Croom Helm.

———. ed. 1981. *Imperialism, Health and Medicine.* Farmingdale, N.Y.: Baywood Publishers.

Newell, K. 1975. *Health by the People.* Geneva: World Health Organization.

Nickel, H. 1980. "The Corporation Haters." *Fortune* 101: 126.

O'Neill, J. 1985. *Five Bodies.* Ithaca, N.Y.: Cornell University Press.

Pasuk Phongpaichit. 1980. *Rural Women of Thailand: From Peasant Girls to Bangkok Masseuses.* Geneva: International Labor Organization.

Peacock, J. 1978. *Purifying the Faith: The Mahammadijah Movement in Indonesian Islam.* Menlo Park, Ca.: Benjamin Cummings Publishing Company.

Pfifferling, J. H. 1981. "A Cultural Prescription for Mediocentrism." In *The Relevance of Social Science for Medicine,* edited by L. Eisenberg and A. Kleinman. Dordrecht: D. Reidel.

Pinckney, C. 1980. "Third World Women and Children Need More Than a Boycott." *Journal of Nurse-Midwifery* 25(3): 25–30.

Post, J. E. 1982. *First World Foods: Third Word Markets. Consumer Issues of the 1980's.* Working Paper, School of Management, Boston University.

———. 1985. "Assessing the Nestlé Boycott: Corporate Accountability and Human Rights." *California Management Review* 27(2): 113–131.

Prentice, A., and R. Pierson. 1982. "Feminism and the Writing and Teaching of History." In *Feminism in Canada,* edited by G. Finn and A. Miles. Montreal: Black Rose Books.

Press, I. 1982. "Witch Doctor's Legacy: Some Anthropological Implications for the Practice of Clinical Medicine." In *Clinically Applied Anthropology,* edited by N. Chrisman and T. Maretzki. Dordrecht: D. Reidel.

Rall, D. 1979. "Foreign Substances in Breast Milk." In *Breastfeeding and Food Policy in a Hungry World,* edited by D. Raphael. New York: Academic Press.

Raphael, D. 1976. *The Tender Gift.* New York: Schocken Books.

———. 1978. "Second Thoughts." *Lactation Review* 3(1): 1.

———. 1981. "Letter to the Editor." *Journal of Nurse-Midwifery* 26(1): 41–43.

———. 1985. *Only Mothers Know.* Westport, Conn.: Greenwood Press.

Richardson, J. L. 1975. "Review of the International Legislation Establishing Nursing Breaks." *Journal of Tropical Pediatrics* 21: 249–258.

Rifkin, S. 1985. *Health Planning and Community Participation.* London: Croom Helm.

Ritenbaugh, C. 1978. "Human Foodways: A Window on Evolution." In *Anthropology of Health,* edited by E. Bauwens. St. Louis: C. V. Mosby Co.

Robinson, K. 1986. "Australia's Got the Milk, We've Got the Problems: The Australian Dairy Corporation in Southeast Asia." In *Shared Wealth and Symbol,* edited by L. Manderson. Cambridge: Cambridge University Press.

Rogers, E. M. 1971. *Communication of Innovations: A Cross Cultural Approach.* New York: Free Press.

———. 1976. "New Product Adoption and Diffusion." *Journal of Consumer Research* (March): 290–301.

Rohde, J. E. 1982. "Mother's Milk and the Indonesian Economy: A Major National Resource." *Journal of Tropical Pediatrics* 28: 166–174.

Rollwagon, J. 1979. "Some Implications of the World System Approach for the Anthropological Study of Latin American Urbanization." *Urban Anthropology* 8(3/4): 249–265.

———. 1980. "New Directions in Urban Anthropology. Building an Ethnography and an Ethnology of the World System." In *Urban Life,* edited by G. Gmelch and W. Zenner. New York: St. Martin's Press.

Rosenberg, H. 1986. "The Kitchen and the Multinational Corporation." In *Through the Kitchen Window,* edited by M. Luxton and H. Rosenberg. Toronto: Garamond Press.

Ross, M., and T. Weisner. 1977. "The Rural-Urban Migrant." *American Ethnologist* 4(2): 359–375.

Rossi, A. 1977. "A Biosocial Perspective on Parenting." *Daedalus* 106: 1–30.

Safilios-Rothschild, C. 1980. "The Role of the Family: A Neglected Aspect of Poverty." World Bank Staff Working Paper, No. 403.

Sansom, B. 1976. "A Signal Transaction and Its Currency." In *Transaction and Meaning,* edited by B. Kapferer. Philadelphia: Institute for the Study of Human Issues.

Savanné, M. A. 1981. "Implications for Women and Their Work of Introducing Nutritional Considerations into Agricultural and Rural Development Projects." *Food and Nutrition Bulletin* 3(3): 1–5.

Scheper-Hughes, N. 1985. "Culture, Scarcity and Maternal Thinking." *Ethos* 13(4): 291–317.

Schumacher, E. F. 1977. *A Guide for the Perplexed.* New York: Harper and Row.

Sen, G., and C. Grown. 1987. *Development, Crises, and Alternative Visions.* New York: Monthly Review Press.

Sharp, L. 1952. "Steel Axes for Stone Age Australians." In

Human Problems in Technological Change, edited by E. Spicer. New York: Russell Sage Foundation.

Short, R. V. 1984. "Breastfeeding." *Scientific American* 250(4): 35–41.

Simpson, M. 1980. "Breastfeeding and Body Contact." *Populi* 7(2): 17–22.

Sommers, M. S. 1986. "Product Symbolism and the Perception of Social Strata." In *Toward Scientific Marketing,* edited by S. A. Greyser. Chicago: A. Mark Associates.

Stacey, J. 1983. "The New Conservative Feminism." *Feminist Studies* 9(3): 559–583.

Stamp, P. 1986. "Kikuyu Women's Self-Help Groups: Toward an Understanding of the Relation between Sex-Gender System and Mode of Production in Africa." In *Women and Class in Africa,* edited by C. Robertson and I. Berger. New York: Africana Publishing Company.

———. 1988. *Gender, Technology and Development in Africa: A Critique of Conceptual Frameworks.* Ottawa: International Development Research Centre.

Steady, F. C. 1981. "Infant Feeding in Developing Countries: Combating the Multinational Imperative." *Journal of Tropical Pediatrics* 27(4): 215–220.

Stoler, A. 1977. "Class Structure and Female Autonomy in Rural Java." *Signs* 3: 74–89.

Stuart-Hagge, P. 1981. "Feminism and Motherhood." *Canadian Society for the Prevention of Cruelty to Children,* Autumn: 3–4.

Sukanya Harntrakul. 1981. "Prostitution and Human Rights in Thailand." *Human Rights in Thailand* (newsletter) 5(3): 5–17.

Sutedjo, M. S 1968. "Nutritional Problems in Indonesia." *Paediatrica Indonesiana* 8: 255–259.

Sutedjo, R. 1974. "Policies and Practices Recommended in Feeding Older Infants and Young Children in Indonesia." *Paediatrica Indonesiana* 14: 185–188.

Svetsreni, T. nd. *Ethnographic Study, Phase Two.* Bangkok: Mahidol University.

Thai Women's Professional Association. 1976. *Reflections of Thai Women*. Bangkok: Thai Kasem Press.

United States Congress. 1978. *Marketing and Promotion of Infant Formula in the Developing Nations*. Washington, D.C.: U.S. Government Printing Office.

Van Esterik, P. 1977. "Lactation, Nutrition, and Changing Cultural Values: Infant Feeding Practices in Rural and Urban Thailand." In *Development and Underdevelopment in Southeast Asia*, edited by G. Means. Ottawa: Canadian Asian Studies Association.

———. 1980a. "The Infant Formula Controversy in Southeast Asia: Advocacy Confrontation or Applied Anthropology?" In *Southeast Asia: Women, Changing Social Structure, and Cultural Continuity*, edited by G. Hainsworth. Ottawa: University of Ottawa Press.

———. 1980b. "Sweetened Condensed Soma: Dietary Innovation in Southeast Asia." *Filipinas: A Journal of Philippine Studies* 1(1): 94–104.

———. 1982. "Infant Feeding Options for Bangkok Professional Women." In *The Decline of the Breast: An Examination of Its Impact on Fertility and health, and Its Relation to Socioeconomic Status*, edited by M. Latham. Cornell International Nutrition Monograph Series, No. 10, Ithaca, N.Y.

———. 1985a. "An Anthropological Perspective on Infant Feeding in Oceania." In *Infant Care and Feeding in Oceania*, edited by L. Marshall. New York: Gordon and Breach.

———. 1985b. "The Cultural Context of Breastfeeding in Rural Thailand." In *Breastfeeding, Child Health and Child Spacing: Cross Cultural Perspectives*, edited by V. Hull and M. Simpson. London: Croom Helm.

———. 1986a. "Confronting Advocacy Confronting Anthropology." In *Advocacy and Anthropology*, edited by R. Paine. St. John's, Newfoundland: Institute of Social and Economic Research.

———. 1986b. "Feeding Their Faith: Recipe Knowledge Among Thai Buddhist Women." *Food and Foodways* 1: 198–215.

———. 1987. "Ideologies and Women in Development Strategies in Thailand." *Proceedings of the International Conference on Thai Studies.* Canberra, Australian National University.

———. 1988. "The Insufficient Milk Syndrome: Biological Epidemic or Cultural Construction?" In *Women and Health: Cross Cultural Perspectives,* edited by P. Whelehan. South Hadley, Mass.: Bergin and Garvey Publishers.

Van Esterik, P., and T. Elliott. 1986. "Infant Feeding Style in Urban Kenya." *Ecology of Food and Nutrition* 18(3): 183–195.

Van Esterik, P., and T. Greiner. 1981. "Breastfeeding and Women's Work: Constraints and Opportunities." *Studies in Family Planning* 12(4): 182–195.

Veblen, T. 1912. *The Theory of the Leisure Class.* New York: Macmillan.

Veldhuis, M., J. Nyamwaya, M. Kinyua, and A. Jansen. 1982. *Knowledge, Attitudes and Practices of Health Workers in Kenya with Respect to Breastfeeding.* Breastfeeding Information Group, Nairobi, Kenya.

Wallerstein, I. 1974. *The Modern World-System: Capitalist Agriculture and the Origins of the European World Economy in the Sixteenth Century.* New York: Academic Press.

Weichert, A. 1975. "Breastfeeding: First Thoughts." *Pediatrics* 56(6): 987–989.

Whitbeck, C. 1984. "A Different Reality: Feminist Ontology." In *Beyond Domination,* edited by C. Gould. Totowa, N.J.: Rowman and Allanheld.

Will, G. 1978. "The Cold War among Women." *Newsweek,* June 26: 100.

Williams, C. 1986. "Milk and Murder." In *Primary Health Care Pioneer. The Selected Works of Dr. Cicely Williams,* edited by N. Baumslay. Geneva: World Federation of Public Health Associations.

Winikoff, B. 1978. "Nutrition, Population and Health: Some Implications for Policy." *Science* 200: 895–902.

Winikoff, B., M. Latham, and G. Solimano. 1983. *The Infant*

Feeding Study: Semarang, Nairobi, Bogotà, and Bangkok Site Reports. New York: Population Council.
Winikoff, B., M. Castle, and V. Laukaran. 1988. *Feeding Infants in Four Societies*. Westport, Conn.: Greenwood Press.
Winzler, R. 1982. "Sexual Status in Southeast Asia: Comparative Perspectives on Women, Agriculture and Political Organization." In *Women of Southeast Asia,* edited by P. Van Esterik. Center for Southeast Asian Studies, Northern Illinois University.
Wipper, A. 1972. "African Women, Fashion and Scapegoating." *Canadian Journal of African Studies* 6(2): 329–349.
Withington, W. 1985. "Indonesia: Insular Contrasts of the Java Core with Outer Islands." In *Southeast Asia: Realm of Contrasts,* edited by A. Dutt. Boulder, Col.: Westview Press.
World Commission on Environment and Development. 1987. *Our Common Future*. New York: Oxford University Press.
World Federation of Public Health Associations. 1986. *Women and Health: Information for Action Issue Paper*. Geneva.
World Health Organization. 1981. *Contemporary Patterns of Breast-Feeding*. Geneva.
Xoomsai, T. 1987. "Bangkok, Thailand: The Quality of Life and Environment in a Primate City." Working Paper No. 48. Joint Centre on Modern East Asia, Toronto.
Zola, I. K. 1972. "Medicine as an Institution of Social Control." *Sociological Review* 20: 487–504.

Index

JOHN RYLANDS
UNIVERSITY
LIBRARY OF
MANCHESTER